Schizophrenia
Schizophrenia

Peter B. Jones MSc, PhD, FRCP, MRCPsych
Professor of Psychiatry and Head of Department,
Department of Psychiatry, University of Cambridge,
Cambridge, UK

Peter F. Buckley MD, MRCPsych
Professor and Chairman,
Department of Psychiatry and Health Behaviour,
Medical College of Georgia,
Augusta, Georgia, USA

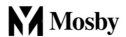

Acknowledgements

The authors wish to acknowledge Soo West for her help in the preparation of this book and the Stanley Medical Research Institute for funding research into the causes of schizophrenia and bipolar disorder.

MOSBY
An imprint of Elsevier Science Limited.

© 2003 Elsevier Science Limited.

The Publisher's policy is to use paper manufactured from sustainable forests

M Mosby is a registered trademark of Elsevier Science Limited.

ISBN 0-7234-3316-X

Cataloguing in Publication Data
Catalogue records for this book are available from the US Library of Congress and the British Library.

Note
Medical knowledge is constantly changing. As new information becomes available, changes in treatment, procedures, equipment and the use of drugs become necessary. The editors/authors/contributors and the publishers have taken care to ensure that the information given in this text is accurate and up to date. However, readers are strongly advised to confirm that the information, especially with regard to drug usage, complies with the latest legislation and standards of practice. All websites correct at time of going to press.

Printed by Grafos S.A. Arte sobre papel, Spain.

Contents

Abbreviations

ACT	assertive community treatment
CBT	cognitive behavioural therapy
CM	case management
DUP	duration of untreated psychosis
DZ	dizygotic
EBM	evidence-based medicine
ECT	electroconvulsive therapy
EPS	extrapyramidal side-effects
fMRI	functional magnetic resonance imaging
HEE	high expressed emotion
MRI	magnetic resonance imaging
MZ	monozygotic
NMDA	*N*-methyl-D-aspartate
NMS	neuroleptic malignant syndrome
OCD	obsessive-compulsive disorder
OR	odds ratio
PET	positron emission tomography
PT	personal therapy
QT_c	QT interval (corrected for heart rate)
QTL	quantitative trait loci
SA	substance abuse co-morbidity
SPD	schizotypal personality disorder
SPET	single photon emission tomography
TR	treatment refractory

Introduction and Background

What is schizophrenia?

A simple question to ask, not such a simple one to answer. If you are going to read and use this book, then you will probably already have a working definition. In fact, a working definition is really all anyone has.

We have to use such a definition carefully, being aware of its limitations and the challenges we accept in using it. We are a long way from really understanding what is and what isn't meant by schizophrenia.

Put at its simplest, schizophrenia is a clinical syndrome, a collection of features that tend to occur together. There is no single most valid definition.[1] Positive psychotic features such as delusions, abnormal thought structure and hallucinations co-occur, in varying degrees if at all, with negative features: the mental, "Parkinsonian" features of restricted emotions, volition and creativity. Even this loose concept isn't good enough, for reasons that will become clear. It is useful, nevertheless, to give some boundaries and to show just how broad and all encompassing this syndrome is when one considers how on earth it might be caused or generated by the mind, and how it might be treated.

As yet there is no accepted aetiological classification of schizophrenia, often seen as the pinnacle of nosology,[2] although suggestions have been made (e.g. familial and sporadic[3]). The disorder exists merely as a clinical syndrome of these symptoms and signs, which is generally useful and which is evolving.[4-6]

In trying to help people and their families, clinicians need some frameworks to give structure to their formulations and plans to intervene and care. Operational criteria for the diagnosis of schizophrenia and related syndromes arose in the middle of the 20th century during an almost terminal bout of self-doubt in psychiatry, the pressures of the anti-psychiatry movement and the contemporary requirements of health insurers. The fourth edition of the *Diagnostic and Statistical Manual* (DSM-IV)[7] and the *International Classification of Diseases*, 10th edition[8] are summaries of the most common, current, clinical ideas on the syndrome (see Tables 1 and 2).

Table 1. DSM-IV: Schizophrenia*

Characteristic symptoms

Two (or more) of the following, each present for a significant portion of time during a 1-month period (or less if successfully treated):

- delusions
- hallucinations
- disorganized speech (e.g. frequent derailment or incoherence)
- grossly disorganized or catatonic behaviour
- negative symptoms, i.e. affective flattening, alogia or avolition

Note: Only one Criterion A symptom is required if delusions are bizarre or hallucinations consist of a voice keeping up a running commentary on the person's behaviour or thoughts, or two or more voices conversing with each other.

Social/occupational dysfunction

For a significant portion of the time since the onset of the disturbance, one or more major areas of functioning such as work, interpersonal relations or self-care are markedly below the level achieved prior to the onset (or when the onset is in childhood or adolescence, failure to achieve expected level of interpersonal, academic or occupational achievement).

*Reprinted with permission from *Diagnostic and Statistical Manual.of Mental Disorder, Fourth Edition*, Text Revision. Copyright 2000 American Psychatric Association.

Table 1 continued. DSM-IV: Schizophrenia*

Duration

Continuous signs of the disturbance persist for at least 6 months. This 6-month period must include at least 1 month of symptoms (or less if successfully treated) that meet Criterion A (i.e. active-phase symptoms) and may include periods of prodromal or residual symptoms. During these prodromal or residual periods, the signs of the disturbance may be manifested by only negative symptoms or two or more symptoms listed in Criterion A present in an attenuated form (e.g. odd beliefs, unusual perceptual experiences).

Schizoaffective and mood disorder exclusion

Schizoaffective disorder and mood disorder with psychotic features have been ruled out because either (1) no major depressive, manic or mixed episodes have occurred concurrently with the active-phase symptoms; or (2) if mood episodes have occurred during active-phase symptoms, their total duration has been brief relative to the duration of the active and residual periods.

Substance/general medical condition exclusion

The disturbance is not due to the direct physiological effects of a substance (e.g. a drug of abuse, a medication) or a general medical condition.

Relationship to a pervasive developmental disorder

If there is a history of autistic disorder or another pervasive developmental disorder, the additional diagnosis of schizophrenia is made only if prominent delusions or hallucinations are also present for at least a month (or less if successfully treated).

Table 1 continued. DSM-IV: Schizophrenia*

Subtypes

295.20 Schizophrenia, Catatonic Type.

295.10 Schizophrenia, Disorganized Type.

295.30 Schizophrenia, Paranoid Type.

295.60 Schizophrenia, Residual Type.

295.90 Schizophrenia, Undifferentiated Type.

Table 2. ICD-10: Schizophrenia (F20)

F20.0–F20.3 General criteria for paranoid, hebephrenic, catatonic and undifferentiated schizophrenia

G1 Either at least one of the syndromes, symptoms and signed listed under (1) below or at least two of the symptoms and signs listed under (2) should be present for most of the time during an episode of psychotic illness lasting for at least 1 month (or at some time during most of the days).

1 At least one of the following must be present:

- thought echo, thought insertion or withdrawal, or thought broadcasting;

- delusions of control, influence or passivity, clearly referred to body or limb movements or specific thoughts, actions or sensations; delusional perception;

- hallucinatory voices giving a running commentary on the patient's behaviour, or discussing the patient between themselves, or other types of hallucinatory voices coming from some part of the body;

- persistent delusions of other kinds that are culturally inappropriate and completely impossible (e.g. being able to control the weather, or being in communication with aliens from another world).

Table 2 continued. ICD-10: Schizophrenia (F20)

2 Or at least two of the following:

- persistent hallucinations in any modality, when occurring every day for at least 1 month, when accompanied by delusions (which may be fleeting or half-formed) without clear affective content, or when accompanied by persistent overvalued ideas;

- neologisms, breaks or interpolations in the train of thought, resulting in incoherence or irrelevant speech;

- catatonic behaviour, such as excitement, posturing or waxy flexibility, negativism, mutism and stupor;

- "negative" symptoms, such as marked apathy, paucity of speech and blunting or incongruity of emotional responses (it must be clear that these are not due to depression or to neuroleptic medication).

G2 Most commonly used exclusion clauses

If the patient also meets the criteria for manic episode (F30) or depressive episode (F32), the criteria listed under G1(1) and G1(2) above must have been met before the disturbance of mood developed.

The disorder is not attributable to organic brain disease (in the sense of F00–F09) or to alcohol- or drug-related intoxication (F1x.0), dependence (F1x.2) or withdrawal (F1x.3 and F1x.4).

Subtypes

F20.1 Hebephrenic schizophrenia.

F20.2 Catatonic schizophrenia.

F20.3 Undifferentiated schizophrenia.

F20.4 Post-schizophrenic depression.

F20.5 Residual schizophrenia.

F20.6 Simple schizophrenia.

F20.8 Other schizophrenia.

F20.9 Schizophrenia unspecified.

Presentation and natural history of schizophrenia: an outline

As can be seen from the diagnostic criteria, the schizophrenia syndrome can have a variety of presentations; it can also run a variable course. This uncertainty about outcome leads commonly to problems in explaining what will happen to those with the syndrome and those who care for them. These problems limit the usefulness of schizophrenia as a diagnosis, and underpin the current habit of referring to *psychosis*. This term is less pejorative and people experience less stigma. It has its original roots in a very broad view of mental disturbance, but is now used to refer to specific symptoms or signs. Those who use the term psychosis need to be more specific about exactly what they mean, in terms of positive symptoms, negative features, social functioning, etc. This is a good thing, but they also need to understand the difference between classification, diagnosis and a full clinical formulation and development of a care plan. People with these disorders are generally most keen on the latter, with an interest in what will happen in the long term; classification is of far less interest to them.

As will become apparent from the later section on the antecedents of schizophrenia, the beginning of the syndrome is often difficult to date, and certainly it is a longitudinal concept, not merely cross-sectional. Schizophrenia is something that develops over time – this means that it might be possible to do something about it sooner rather than later. Criteria such as the DSM-IV are couched in terms of an active phase of largely psychotic symptoms and a preceding, "prodromal" phase of less specific phenomena. Certainly, the longer one is required to be ill before meeting criteria, the worse the outcome is likely to be for a person who does.

Features of the prodromal period include withdrawal from previous social roles, impairment in general functioning, behaviour others see as odd, altered emotions (blunted affect or inappropriateness), deterioration in personal hygiene, difficulties communicating with others, strange ideas, unusual perceptual experiences, and restricted drive, initiative, interests or energy.

These features are often summed up by others as the person "not being themselves"; people in a prodrome will sometimes say that "something is not quite right". The duration of the prodrome variable and its onset may be difficult to date. Sometimes, the onset is insidious and it may not be possible to identify a true change, particularly in younger people who will be changing anyway, as part of their normal development. In such cases, the loss of function and the more general concept of "social capital" can be profound. The prodome in these people will be developing just as they should be consolidating their education, occupational roles and adult relationships.

One can see how the process of development of schizophrenia may evolve, and with it the diagnosis. One modern view of schizophrenia is that of an *outcome* of a process. There often appears to be continuity between premorbidly abnormal personality, insidious onset, disabling negative symptoms and poor outcome; some believe that this continuity is mediated by the cognitive deficits discussed later. However, the differential diagnosis of negative symptoms must always be borne in mind, because interventions, that may be very effective, differ (Table 3).

Even when there is a clear change, it should be remembered that the prodrome, despite its name, is an entirely retrospective concept. We know definitely that a collection of suspicious and disabling features occur as a prodrome to schizophrenia once the schizophrenia syndrome has emerged, but there is much less certainty beforehand; features early in the prodrome may be very non-specific. As in other situations, we can be much more certain about the future after it has happened than before.

Early interventions

In addition to variability in the length of the prodrome, the length of time of active psychosis can vary greatly, commonly being measured in months or even years before people seek or get help. The reasons vary. This phase, or *duration of untreated psychosis*, is referred to as DUP.

The length of the DUP does appear to be related to outcome; the longer the DUP, the worse the prognosis. The mechanism

Table 3. Differential diagnosis and management of apparent negative features

Negative feature	Intervention
Depression	Antidepressant medication and psychological intervention such as cognitive therapy
Positive symptoms paradoxically leading to inactivity (e.g. running commentary hallucinations quelled only by inactivity)	Review antipsychotic drug regimen and consider cognitive or other psychological intervention
Extrapyramidal syndrome* thereafter	Review antipsychotic regimen,and be very carefu
True negative symptons	Review antipsychotic regimen and whole care plan, including occupational therapy and social aspects

*This may also be a feature at presentation; extrapyramidal features occur in drug-naive people.

Table 4. Possible causes or mediators of long DUP and poor outcome

Neurobiological toxicity, with neural activity underlying psychosis strengthening neural networks – akin to *kindling*

Psychological trauma of frightening psychotic phenomena leading to features of post-traumatic stress disorder

Accrual of disabilities during untreated phase. The longer young people are ill, the further behind they fall in terms of education, occupation and social role development

Continuity of other factors such as abnormal premorbid personality, insidious onset, cognitive deficits and negative features. These drive poor outcome and, incidentally, lead to longer DUP

is not clear; there are a number of possible, or alternative, explanations (Table 4).

Further research is needed in order to decide which of these factors regarding DUP is most important, but it is possible that several or even all play a role. Certainly, many professional disciplines and most who use services can identify with one or several explanations. This may be helping to drive the expansion of specialist *early intervention* services aimed at first-episode psychosis, trying to reduce the DUP (Table 5); they are not necessarily aimed only at young people.

Clearly, it is important to identify people with psychosis as soon as possible after the onset of positive psychotic symptoms. A public health aim would, reasonably, be to identify people before they became psychotic, so long as there were interventions with an acceptable risk : benefit ratio. However, methods of prediction are not yet adequate for this kind of screening to warrant the false positives; even careful follow-up would not necessarily be benign for these people who would, no doubt, be alarmed. However, situations 3 and 4 in Table 5 certainly are the proper remit of services. Even if we cannot reliably identify prodromes without false positives, those who contact services with changed mental states are morbid and require help, regardless of whether they will develop psychosis. Trials in these situations are ongoing and important.[9] Situation 5 in Table 5 should now be obsolete in modern services. McGorry[10] has provided many excellent reviews of these issues and pioneering services in Australia.

Table 5. Interpretations of "early intervention" in psychosis
Before there is any sign of change or illness – primary prevention in the general population
Defining people at high risk but before there are overt signs of psychosis
Intervening in people with problems or "*At Risk Mental States*" who have made contact with services and, perhaps, are seen by a specialist service
Prompt, proper interventions for first-episode psychotic syndromes
Avoiding long delays in the delivery of effective intervention, care or rehabilitation in established schizophrenia

Following an initial manic or psychotic syndrome, about 40% will either never meet criteria for schizophrenia, having either long-term affective syndromes or non-affective diagnoses defined by their brief course, or their cause (such a drug intoxication).

For those who develop the schizophrenia syndrome, a residual or stable phase often follows the acute phase of the illness and the initiation of treatment. The features of this phase will often resemble the prodrome, frequently with some residual, attenuated psychotic phenomena that should be rigorously treated. However, emotional blunting or flattening and impairment in social role functioning is common.

The typical course is one of acute exacerbation, possibly precipitated by stress, illicit drug use, non-compliance with maintenance treatment, or a combination of these. There may be residual impairment between episodes. However, this course can be changed a great deal by the degree and quality of intervention provided, and is very variable between individuals.

Evidence from the WHO Ten Country Study and elsewhere suggests that after 2–3 years this course will become clear, and that this period may be a key period to get things right. Certainly, all concerned must remain optimistic during this initial period and focus efforts on making it more likely that the person concerned will have minimal residual symptoms or social impairment.

Only some predictors of outcome are fixed (see Table 6). The nub of the early psychosis paradigm is to alter all malleable predictors, to engage people early in the assessment of their needs in a broad sense, to maximize the effectiveness of all interventions that are used, and to stick at it. The aim is to minimize impairment and promote recovery.

Social functioning and outcome

Schizophrenia involves impairment in many domains, often over and above the direct effect of positive psychotic features. Thus, one can describe a variety of disabilities that may affect someone with the disorder. The schema in Table 7 arose during the development of rehabilitation psychiatry, but remains useful if recent concepts are added.

Table 6. Predictors of good outcome in schizophrenia

Female gender

Later age at onset – there is no threshold

Acute onset, often with apparent confusion

Precipitating factors or life events

Normal pre-psychotic personality

Good social, educational and occupational functioning

No negative features

No cognitive impairment

No family history of schizophrenia

Affective features or family history of affective disorder

Effective interventions maintained without side-effects

Not having the features of schizophrenia for long – a truism, but underlines the element of chronicity, and so poorer prognosis, built into the criteria

Table 7. Disabilities and impairments in schizophrenia – a conceptual framework

Primary disabilities	• Positive and negative psychotic features
	• Depression and other psychopathology
	• Drug side-effects
	• Cognitive dysfunction
Secondary disabilities	• Loss of social capital
	• Education
	• Family
	• Friends
	• Occupational opportunity
	• Independence and esteem
Tertiary disabilities	• Results of stigma
	• Loss of opportunities
	• Discrimination

Impairments arise as a result of primary and, to some extent, tertiary disabilities (Figure 1). They include occupational functioning, social relations and looking after oneself on a

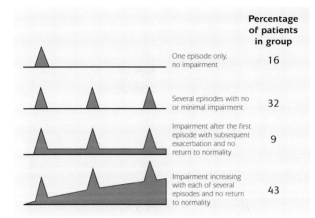

		Percentage of patients in group
	One episode only, no impairment	16
	Several episodes with no or minimal impairment	32
	Impairment after the first episode with subsequent exacerbation and no return to normality	9
	Impairment increasing with each of several episodes and no return to normality	43

Figure 1. Five-year outcome following a first presentation of schizophrenia. Services should aim to shift everyone up this caricature of outcome. Overall, we would hope to be doing somewhat better now than these figures indicate, but this shows the range of outcomes. Reproduced with permission of Cambridge University Press from *The Recognition and Management of Early Psychosis*, edited by McGorry PD, Jackson HJ, 1999. This was originally adapted from Shepherd M. *et al*. The natural history of schizophrenia: a five year follow up and prediction in a representative sample of schizophrenics. *Psychol Med* Monograph Supplement 1989: **15**: 1–46.[11]

day-to-day level. This impairment varies across the different phases of the disorder, and is by no means always related to positive symptoms. Negative symptoms and cognitive problems are the key determinants, particularly when positive features are less potent for an individual, something that can be achieved with drug and psychological interventions, even when the phenomena themselves remain present. Certainly, they are more amenable to intervention than issues like society's attitudes to mental illness.

Some people may require supervision to ensure adequate nutrition and hygiene standards, and to protect the person from the consequences of impulsivity, poor judgement, cognitive impairment, or acting in response to delusional beliefs or command hallucinations. Between episodes of illness, the extent of residual disability may range from none to significant levels.

Violence by people with schizophrenia attracts media and public attention, and may influence health policy in a remarkably direct way. While the frequency of such acts is marginally higher than in the general population, this will be the same for many comparison groups and the absolute rates remain very low. Normal human psychology, particularly in men, is responsible for a far greater toll, and the risk in the population attributable to alcohol and other drug misuse is far higher than to any mental illness. The combination of positive features of schizophrenia, drug abuse and loss of contact with services and treatments is, however, a combination that services should aim to avoid.

The life expectancy of people with schizophrenia is shorter than that of the general population. An important cause is suicide, with approximately 10% dying in this way; suicide prevention is another important aspect of any care plan. Accelerated mortality from a variety of other causes makes physical care and health promotion (including sexual health and drug advice) a vital consideration from first onset.

Some history of the concept and further thoughts about schizophrenia

As a "functional" psychosis, the syndrome is often defined as being without cause, or at least one thought of as acting on the brain rather than the psyche.[12] Known causes of the syndrome, such as some drugs and epilepsies, lead to a diagnosis being excluded in contemporary classifications, including the two used here, and in the most recent major classifications used for research – namely, DSM-IV and ICD-10 referred to in this book. This is ridiculous.

The harmful effect that this persistence of a Cartesian mind–body split may have on the search for the causes of schizophrenia is well recognized.[3, 13] It does not rest easily with contemporary, neurobiological formulations of the mechanisms of normal and abnormal mental phenomena. We won't explore reductionist arguments,[14] but any good explanation of any psychological event cannot be thought of as complete unless brain function (or dysfunction) is included. A theory of schizophrenia has to explain everything about the disorder if it is to be complete. However, an incomplete explanation can still be a useful one, one explaining delusions or difficulties in social functioning, for instance.

Some features of the schizophrenia syndrome can be recognized in classical Greek literature.[15] The Ancients considered them to be separate from the agitations or manic states which were accompanied by fever, conditions they called the "phrenitides". This is similar to the distinction, mentioned above, that some still make today between functional and organic psychosis, something that may be holding back our understanding (see below). Keeping at a clinical level, it was during the 19th century that nosologists and physicians began to group together these syndromes not associated with manifest organic states (such as general paralysis of the insane or neurosyphilis) into distinct mental disorders.

Dementia praecox
Kraepelin (Figure 2) is widely credited with the first description of what would today be recognized as

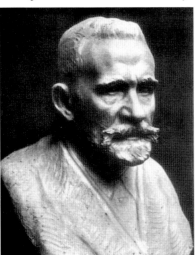

Figure 2. Emil Kraepelin 1856–1926, an enormously influential German psychiatrist, himself influenced by the experimental psychology of Wilhelm Wundt. A concise biography of Kraepelin can be found at http://www.uni-leipzig.de/~psy/eng/kraep-e.html. Photo courtesy of Royal College of Psychiatrists.

schizophrenia,[16] as well as having developed a number of modern clinical psychiatric practices and an experimental approach to understanding psychology. Kraepelin used the term "dementia praecox" to subsume the syndromes of catatonia, hebephrenia and dementia paranoides into a single entity within the functional, "endogenous" psychoses. Kraepelin distinguished this group from manic depression and from the dementia associated with old age, which he later named Alzheimer's disease in recognition of the contribution to its characterization by his friend and colleague. Depression and melancholia were already considered as separate. Kraepelin's first description of dementia praecox was published in 1896 in the fifth edition of his textbook, *Psychiatrie*,[17] refined 3 years later in the sixth edition. This is usually read in the eighth edition,[18] when he had included in the definition the "dementia simplex" described by Pick[19] and by Diem.[20]

However, the term dementia praecox used in this way did not arise out of the blue; it was based on other descriptions of the 19th century. Pinel[21] had used "demence" to describe psychotic states, and Morel[22, 23] used the term "demence precoce" when he reported psychosis beginning in the teenage years. Snell[24] had already separated primary paranoid states (*primare Verrucktheit*) from mania and melancholia, Kahlbaum[25] had distinguished catatonia, and Hecker[26] had described the phenomenology of hebephrenia, a description upon which Kraepelin drew later in his first, 1896, account. These authors tended to view these states as separate entities until Fink[27] described mixed states of catatonia and hebephrenia. Kraepelin further described the phenomenology and clinical characteristics of dementia praecox, but stressed the young age at onset and deteriorating course as the major distinguishing features of dementia praecox.

Schizophrenia

Twelve years after Kraepelin's first account, Eugene Bleuler (Figure 3) questioned both these characteristics when he outlined his views of the prognosis of dementia praecox.[28] He

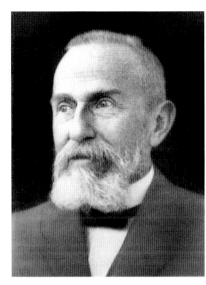

Figure 3. Eugene Bleuler, Swiss psychiatrist and psychologist. Born 30 April 1857, Zollikon near Zürich, died 15 July 1939, Zollikon. Photo courtesy of Royal College of Psychiatrists.

felt that the splitting or tearing apart of the psychic functions that occurred in the disorder was a more unifying characteristic than either age at onset or deteriorating course (although he acknowledged the view that the syndrome did usually deteriorate). Having written with touching deference in his text to Kraepelin's contribution, he went on to use the term "*Schizophreniegruppe*", the group of schizophrenias, to describe this. The first part of this term has stuck and is best described in a later account.[29]

Bleuler stressed the phenomena of a disintegration of personality, with disturbances of formulation and expression of thinking. Perception and the sense of reality were altered, and there was an incongruous affect. He considered that these were common to a group of heterogeneous psychotic conditions that could occur in clear consciousness without obvious brain disease. In the 1911 account, Bleuler also divided these phenomena into the primary or fundamental psychological dysfunctions of altered associations (disordered thought form and structure), altered affect, ambivalence and autism, and the secondary features such as delusions and hallucinations that he considered to be the result of, or secondary to, the primary features.

Bleuler intended to narrow the concept of schizophrenia by emphasizing these underlying or primary features; he considered delusions and hallucinations as non-specific. The opposite happened, possibly due to the emerging *Zeitgeist* of psychoanalysis.[30] Bleuler's primary disturbances were difficult to define specifically and were seen widely by psychiatrists in their patients' states of mind. Attention is drawn to them here because they infer the notion that several systems of the mind and brain are disturbed in schizophrenia, and that such disturbances may exist independently of the more dramatic phenomena that are stressed in descriptions of the clinical syndrome, e.g. hallucinations. Minkowski[31] summarized the views of others[32] and incorporated his own into a view of schizophrenia (although he still called it dementia praecox) as a disorder of the harmonious interplay between several mental functions. This view is regaining popularity, particularly as explained by a mechanism of disordered neural connectivity (see below). It underlies the approach taken here to examine the thesis in terms of risk factors reflecting, and possibly affecting, several psycho-logical and brain systems, both at the time of psychosis and before it begins.

The schizophrenia concept continued to develop over subsequent decades, yielding rather than culminating in the current, operational, clinical definitions, although the concept is more fluid in many areas of research (discussed by Castle and Murray[33]), concentrating on individual symptoms rather than the syndrome. The modern definitions owe a lot to the phenomenological school, particularly regarding positive psychotic phenomena.

Kurt Schneider was central to steering definitions towards an exclusively phenomenological one when he published a list of the symptoms that he considered to be of first-rank importance (Table 8), or most useful when trying to make a diagnosis of schizophrenia.[34] Other symptoms he considered as less discriminatory, or of second-rank importance.

Table 8. Symptoms that Schneider considered of first-rank importance

Hearing your thoughts spoken aloud

Hearing voices talking about you – third person hallucinations

Hearing a voice(s) describing what you're doing (running commentary)

Somatic hallucinations

Thought withdrawal and/or insertion

Thought broadcasting

Delusional perception

Feelings or actions made, controlled or influenced by forces outside the self

With the addition of criteria for altered social functioning and chronicity, and exclusion criteria such as predominating depression and organic brain conditions, these first-rank symptoms form the basis of the modern operational definitions, though none is necessary or specific. Schneider himself was rather modest in describing his list, suggesting that it might help the diagnosis of schizophrenia, not shape the concept for decades to come.

These modern operational classifications (so-called diagnostic menus) followed the demonstration in the early 1970s of unacceptable discrepancies in definitions of schizophrenia used by English and American psychiatrists.[35] This work precipitated the development and widespread use of operational diagnostic criteria, now available across the spectrum of psychiatric conditions. The trap of mistaking reliability for validity in these definitions is well recognized,[1] but they have made much research evidence at least reliable, or more comparable between studies.

All operational systems rely on a largely cross-sectional definition of schizophrenia as a clinical syndrome. The core features are certain types of auditory hallucinations, particularly voices heard talking in the third person, changes in thought construction and form and, finally, bizarre delusions which often involve a person's ego boundary, such that thoughts may be available to others or a person is influenced by outside forces.

These *positive*, psychotic phenomena, comprising the core diagnostic features, are heavily influenced by Schneider's ideas. They usually occur together with changes in an individual's behaviour or social functioning. There may also be so-called *negative* features, such as restriction of the range of emotions and decreased ability to initiate thoughts and ideas; these are Kraepelin's and Bleuler's legacy, recently developed further by Andreasen. Some criteria, such as the early DSM, incorporate items regarding short-term course, something which may have a major impact on research into outcomes, and even on aetiological research, where predisposing and precipitating factors may be confused with those that perpetuate the disorder.[36]

None of the core features of schizophrenia is pathognomonic, although the presence of at least one, in the absence of an obvious organic precipitant, such as drug misuse, is essential for the diagnosis. As Bleuler proposed, several psychological systems can be affected, including perceptions in various modalities, the generation, construction and inferential use of thoughts, emotions and volition.

Andreasen[1] has summarized her own and others' views of schizophrenia as it approached its centenary. She emphasized the polythetic nature of schizophrenia and the division of its features into positive and negative, along the lines suggested originally by Jackson[37] and later by Crow.[38] Andreasen notes that the array of signs and symptoms classified as positive or negative is often summarized according to the range of cognitive and emotional domains involved. Overall, schizophrenia must involve many brain systems or sub-systems (Table 9).

There are two competing explanations in anatomical terms. On the assumption that the functions and systems in Table 10 can each be localized to specific brain regions, the first suggests that schizophrenia may be a condition such as multiple sclerosis or cerebral lupus, where multiple, discrete lesions in different sites produce a varied and heterogeneous condition.[39, 40] The second, again reminiscent of Bleuler, Stransky and Minkowski, draws upon ideas of distributed parallel processing.[39,41] Abnormalities of the connectivity or "wiring" of the brain may produce multiple effects depending upon the circuits involved

Table 9. Relationship between features of schizophrenia and neural systems

Symptom	Neural system or sub-system
Positive	
Hallucinations	Perception
Delusions	Inferential thinking
Disorganized speech/thought form	Language
Disorganized/bizarre behaviour/catatonia	Behavioural monitoring and secondary to other psychotic phenomena
Negative	
Alogia	Conceptual fluency
Affective blunting	Emotional expression
Anhedonia	Experiencing pleasure
Avolition	Volition
Other	
Motor signs at onset	Extrapyramidal and other motor systems
Cognitive deficits	Wide range of cortical and sub-cortical systems

The diagnosis of affective psychosis versus schizophrenia rests largely on the single affective item that can have a range of expression other than blunting in other disorders, and in schizophrenia as well. The multiplicity of systems affected suggests to many an underlying difference in integrative or connectivity mechanisms.

and the site of the problem. The complexity of brain circuitry would ensure a multiplicity of inter-related symptoms[42, 43] and other cognitive effects manifest only with specific tests.

Since the early 1970s, this latter idea of disordered functional connectivity in schizophrenia has been amenable to direct investigation by functional neuroimaging techniques, first[44] by crude, single photon emission tomography (SPET), and now by high-resolution SPET, positron emission tomography (PET) and functional magnetic resonance imaging (fMRI). Cognitive tasks, such as verbal fluency, are used to activate and suppress activity in specific cortical areas, and normal subjects are compared with those with schizophrenia in terms of space and time.[45] As originally suggested by Wernike,[46] a disturbance of connections between the prefrontal and temporal cortices would fit many clinical data concerning schizophrenia. Recent ideas concerning causation might also fit in with such a model, including the timing of possible aetiological events in mid-pregnancy,[47–49] when relevant connections are being formed.[50] These ideas are considered again in the section on causes.

McGuire and Frith[51] noted that the direct evidence for *dys*connectivity in schizophrenia is as yet largely circumstantial, "its popularity owing as much to conceptual appeal as it does to scientific data". However, there is an opportunity to test, in biological terms, the model put forward by Bleuler. The field is reviewed by Friston.[52]

These ideas ignore many other attempts, particularly in continental Europe (see Hirsch and Shepherd[53] for a review), to identify and define the clinical borders of schizophrenia within mental illness. The review here has stressed the widespread nature of the psychopathology in the clinical syndrome even when this is defined narrowly by modern criteria. The syndrome is a cross-sectional one, but may be better thought of in longitudinal terms, with the clinical syndrome and its subsequent course as part of its evolution;[48] this influences modern practices in terms of diagnosis and underpins the contemporary early intervention movement.

In terms of the brain and mind, what we call schizophrenia could alternatively be regarded as the *effects* of schizophrenia, not a disease in itself. If so, then the true definition of schizophrenia remains almost as elusive as it has been over the rest of the century, but at least we know where to look, in the structure and functioning of the brain, as well as the phenomena it generates.

Problems with categorical definitions and operational criteria

One fundamental problem concerns aetiology, or rather the lack of it, in our definitions. Medicine likes to classify disease on the basis of cause and mechanism. We mustn't be too hard on psychiatry for not adopting this stance, because we are unsure of the true causes and mechanisms for many psychiatric disorders, except for those where this forms part of the definition, such as post-traumatic stress disorder. Here, building a cause into the definition means that we assume the category is distinct from other anxiety disorders, and we can't be certain of that either. Not being able to find causes or genetic linkage also shakes faith in the current schizophrenia concepts.

However, we do a strange thing with schizophrenia in that whenever we have a possible *organic* cause for the syndrome, like epilepsy, we say this isn't schizophrenia. We've become paralysed by the old idea of schizophrenia as a *functional* psychosis and rule out the diagnosis when there is gross neuropathology or brain disease. This is despite the accumulating evidence (and common sense view) that there is an underlying neurobiological substrate for the production of these features.

Another problem concerns the boundaries, not between different psychotic syndromes, although these overlap, co-exist or evolve in interesting ways, but between normality and psychosis. Psychologists have long been interested in personality dimensions in psychosis, such as schizotypy, that may share some genetic causes with schizophrenia, and in cognitive vulnerability. Recent psychiatric and epidemiological interest has quickened, particularly due to the work of van Os and Verdoux, who have shown not only that individual psychotic symptoms (not the syndrome) are relatively common in young adults, but that they share some of the same risk factors and, perhaps, causes. The point is illustrated in Figure 4, showing results from the Epidemiological Catchment Area programme[54] (ECA). Individual psychotic symptoms were remarkably common in the general population of North America.

Cognition and neuropsychology

We are left with a syndrome where loss of function over a period of time, often leading to contact with health services, assumes considerable importance when defining whether someone with symptoms has schizophrenia, is within normal limits, or has a psychotic syndrome within the penumbra of the schizophrenias.

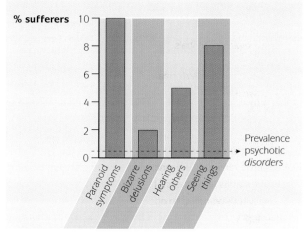

Figure 4. Prevalence of psychotic symptoms in the general population. Adapted from Eaton *et al.*[55]

Table 10. Organic or functional? A comprehensive review of neuropsychological classifications of schizophrenic versus brain damaged
94 studies between 1960 and 1975. Heaton, Baade and Johnson, *Psychol Bull* 1978; **85**: 141–162[56]
50% classification on the basis of neuropsychology is chance
For chronic schizophrenia (34 cases) there was only 54% correct classification – just about chance levels
Schizophrenia and brain damage appeared the same on the basis of neuropsychology in these studies during a period when some said schizophrenia was a myth

Kraepelin and Bleuler were both well versed in the experimental and cognitive psychology of their time, and emphasized underlying mechanisms in these spheres. The ideas went out of fashion in the middle of the 20th century, as psychodynamic formulations clouded the search for the causes of schizophrenia. Even so, as we have seen above, studies on

Table 11. What is the range of neuropsychological deficits?

Event-related potentials

Sustained attention
- The Continous Performance Task

Selective attention

Memory
- Explicit>implicit, recall and recognition
- Working memory – dorsolateral prefrontal cortex (DLPFC)

Executive functions – planning and set-shifting

fMRI suggests less efficient frontal lobe function

General IQ – one-third to one-half a standard deviation

Psychophysiology

general function, or IQ, were regularly showing a deficit in people with schizophrenia and, in fact, evidence of neuropsychological problems as severe as in acquired brain damage was present in the literature (see Table 10).

Over the past decade there has been a burgeoning of interest in neuropsychological deficits in schizophrenia, their relationship to symptoms and outcome, how they may map onto underlying neural systems, and how they may be manipulated (Table 11). This last issue is of particular interest, as there is substantial evidence for a strong link between neurocognitive deficits and poor functional outcome in schizophrenia (Figure 5).[57] Interventions that could improve cognition would be helpful.

Attention, memory and executive functions are particularly implicated, with systems involving the dorsolateral prefrontal cortex important. It is likely that the continuity of abnormal premorbid personality, insidious onset, negative symptoms and poor outcome are all manifestations of the same underlying deficit, perhaps changing with maturity of the relevant neural systems, and perhaps reflecting genetic and epigenetic processes described later in the section on causes.

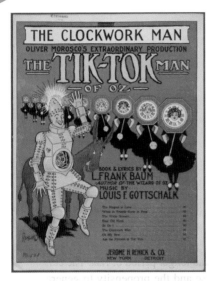

Figure 5. Neuropsychological mechanisms of psychosis and outcome are topical, and may represent the endo-phenotype in schizophrenia and other psychoses. They may also be the substrate upon which genetic risk has its action, amongst many other candidates. There may not be a single, vulnerable cognition or deficit, but a range of otherwise adaptive cognitive patterns may pose a risk of psychosis when they occur together. This is akin to genetic models involving multiple genes of small effect. Interested readers should consult a specialist reference.

Epidemiology

Who gets schizophrenia?

Age

The safest answer is that anyone can get this syndrome. However, there are two remarkably constant findings in the epidemiology of schizophrenia. The first is that it tends to have its onset in young adulthood, being extremely rare before puberty. The figures from landmark studies by Slater and Cowie in the 1960s and by Häfner *et al.*[58] a quarter of a century later summarize the situation (Figure 6). They also demonstrate the slight difference between men and women, who tend to have a somewhat later onset and longer period of risk. The close link between the life-course and the propensity to generate the schizophrenia syndrome probably betrays an underlying neurobiological phenomenon, such as the maturation of certain connections through normal or abnormal myelination.

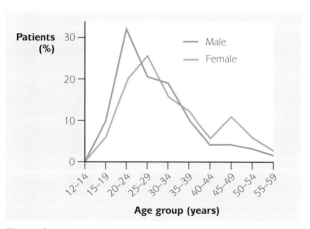

Figure 6. Age at onset of schizophrenia. Reproduced with permission from Häfner H, Riescher-Rossler A, An Der Heiden W *et al*. Generating and testing a causal explanation of the gender differences in age at first onset of schizophrenia. *Psychol Med* 1993; **23**(4): 925–940.[58]

Gender

The second consistent finding is that the disorder is rather more common in men when it is tightly defined in terms of excluding affective symptoms. Most studies with modern criteria include as few as half as many women as men in the first half of life, with the balance being restored later on. This increased incidence in women in later life, independently of dementia, may hold aetiological clues, with oestrogen systems implicated as protectors before the menopause.

When does schizophrenia really begin?

The data on age at onset demonstrate that the emergence of the schizophrenia syndrome is intimately related to the life-course, and in an unusual way. In general, most pathological processes occur at the extremes of life, but schizophrenia occupies this intermediate position. This accounts, in part, for its huge personal, familial, social and economic impact.

Evidence of developmental differences is difficult to refine regarding those who will later become psychotic and those who will not. Kraepelin[17] and Bleuler[28, 29] both noticed that a considerable proportion of people who developed the psychotic syndrome of schizophrenia had been different, in terms of character and behaviour, during childhood and youth.

Their astute clinical observations were possible because they were, in large part, informally observing their patients' children before some developed illnesses similar to their parents. Thus, they made opportunistic use of genetic high-risk and cohort designs. However, the inference that the remainder of those who would develop schizophrenia had entirely *normal* development may not be justified.

Much of the evidence for abnormal development prior to psychosis, such as from studies of minor physical anomalies and neuropathology, is *best* (but not necessarily completely) explained in terms of developmental processes having gone wrong.[59] However, these processes are not observed directly. Genetic high-risk studies have shown subtle differences in neurological development in high-risk children.[60–63]

General population and genetic high-risk studies are two key tools. The evidence is convergent between the two research paradigms. General population cohorts can be considered as another type of high-risk paradigm where the children who will develop schizophrenia are at 100% risk, and are compared with their peers at zero risk.

High-risk studies

Developmental abnormalities throughout childhood have been found in one-quarter to one-half of "high-risk" children who are born to mothers with schizophrenia.[61, 64] These include:

- hypoactivity;
- hypotonia and poor "cuddliness" during the neonatal period;
- an unusual pattern and slow attainment of milestones in infancy;
- "soft" neurological signs, in particular poor motor co-ordination in early childhood;
- deficits in attention and information processing in late childhood.

These findings indicate that at least part of the genetic vulnerability to schizophrenia involves, or is accompanied by, abnormal neurodevelopment. Attention and other cognitive deficits are likely to be of key importance.

Early milestones and motor development in general population studies

There is direct evidence of neurodevelopmental differences in children who will get schizophrenia as adults. Elaine Walker and colleagues[63] studied "home movies" of families in which one child later developed schizophrenia. They rated emotion and motor function blind to that child's identity amongst their siblings. The children who would as adults develop schizophrenia were distinguished on both accounts. Some remarkable, but transitory, motor differences were clear.

Similar developmental differences have now been demonstrated in several epidemiological samples from around the world.

In the British 1946 birth cohort (the Medical Research Council National Survey of Health and Development, NSHD; Wadsworth[65, 66]), the first of the long-term, birth cohort studies in the UK, a range of childhood developmental differences were found.[67] Milestones were assessed by maternal recall at age 24 months, and all those recorded, sitting, standing, walking and talking, were delayed. There were indications that language development was different in these children. Health visitors were more likely to notice no speech by 2 years in the children who developed schizophrenia as adults, and school doctors noted speech delays and problems throughout childhood.

These developmental differences have been replicated in other cohorts. The British 1958 cohort (the National Child Development Study, NCDS) is the second of the three British birth cohorts and involves all children born in the same week as the NSHD, but 12 years later. Pre-schizophrenia children at age 7 had been slower to develop continence, and had poor co-ordination and vision. At age 16 they were rated clumsy.[68, 69]

Cannon et al.[70] studied a cohort of births in Helsinki between 1951 and 1960, linking birth and school records to the Finnish Hospital Discharge Register. Children who had schizophrenia as adults were rated at school as having problems with sports and handicrafts. This may be a manifestation of the same unco-ordinated motor characteristics as Crow et al.[68] demonstrated, and of the delayed milestones noted in the earlier British cohort.[71]

Two recent studies leave the existence of these subtle developmental abnormalities beyond doubt. The North Finland 1966 birth cohort involved all 12,000 children due to be born in northern Finland during 1966.[72] Isohanni et al.[73] have indicated that the developmental differences are present even in the first year of life. There was evidence of a dose–response relationship between the age at which a boy could stand or walk without support, and his risk of subsequent schizophrenia; the later he walked, the more likely he was to develop schizophrenia (Figure 7).

Not walking unsupported at age 1 is by no means abnormal, the absolute size of these effects is small, and schizophrenia

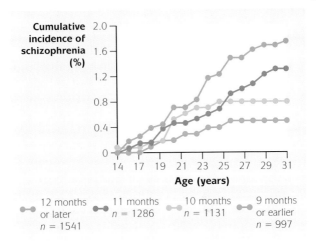

Cumulative incidence of schizophrenia (%)

Age (years)

12 months or later
n = 1541

11 months
n = 1286

10 months
n = 1131

9 months or earlier
n = 997

Figure 7. The later a boy learned to stand during the first year of life, the greater was his risk of schizophrenia a decade or two later. Reproduced from Isohanni M et al. Early developmental milestones in adult schizophrenia and other psychoses. A 31-year follow-up of the North Finland 1966 birth cohort. *Schizophrenia Res* 2001; **52**: 1–19[73] with permission from Elsevier Science.

is not solely a disorder of motor development. However, a dose–response relationship is a very potent finding in epidemiology, and the important thing about this one is that it operates within the normal range. Subjects who would later develop schizophrenia may have been walking just a little later than they might have been had they not have been subject to some pathological process that increased the risk of schizophrenia. It is not helpful to consider those who were late walkers in terms of being well below the mean as being at particular, or different, risk compared with the rest of the children who developed schizophrenia.

The latest results regarding early maturational effects before schizophrenia come from the Dunedin birth cohort study, in which continuity between self-reported psychotic experiences in childhood and a fairly broad concept of schizophreniform disorder arising by the early twenties has been reported recently.[74] Cannon *et al.*[75] have demonstrated similarly

Table 12. Summary of developmental differences prior to adult schizophrenia seen in the general population

Later motor development milestones

More speech problems during childhood

Evidence of failure of integrative development and presence of soft signs

Lower educational test scores during childhood and adolescence

Preference for solitary play

Anxiety in social situations and sometimes problems with conduct

widespread developmental delays in several modalities before schizophreniform disorder, these being rather specific to this disease category.

These subtle effects have become one of the most replicated findings in the developmental epidemiology of schizophrenia over the past decade. Each of the remarkable studies that have been investigated brings a slightly different view of the phenomenon. Regardless of their small size, these developmental differences are likely to betray biologically significant processes relevant to the development of schizophrenia (Table 12). They also indicate that causal processes were already active in very early life. It seems that the differences were most apparent "on the cusp" of developmental processes. Grown up, the children did not have gross motor or speech problems, although psychosis and the motor aspects of the schizophrenia syndrome[76] may be the later manifestations of the same mechanism(s), with the study by Poulton et al.[74] indicating hitherto unrecognized continuity of psychopathology. Kraepelin described motor problems in people with schizophrenia half a century before antipsychotic medication was described. We are just beginning to relearn their significance.

Behavioural development

Studies of behaviour have also evolved from early clinical accounts. Retrospective assessment of behaviour and personality demonstrate differences prior to psychosis, with the most common being characteristics of a rather shy, schizoid habit.[77–80]

Robins[81] carried out a pioneering, historical cohort study in which she followed a group of boys who had been referred to a child guidance clinic. Antisocial behaviour was associated with later schizophrenia in this sample. Watt and Lubensky[82, 83] traced the school records of cases of schizophrenia from a geographically defined neighbourhood in Massachusetts. Girls who were later to develop schizophrenia were introverted throughout kindergarten into adolescence. Boys in the same predicament were "disagreeable", but only in the later school grades (7–12). Done *et al.*[84] have identified a remarkably similar behavioural pattern in the British 1958 birth cohort, including the changes over time. "Schizoid" behavioural differences are seen in the British 1946 cohort,[85] and in two large studies of conscripts in Sweden[86] and Israel.[87, 88]

Given current views (again relearning what Kraepelin and Bleuler already thought) concerning the cognitive disturbances that accompany, and may underpin, psychosis, it seems a reasonable and parsimonious hypothesis that the early developmental and behavioural effects may be linked through cognition.[89] The motor and language findings betray a disturbance or difference in developmental processes. This is manifest in behavioural terms because the same processes affect cognitive development, particularly in the realm of social cognition. Any difference in behaviour and interaction with others may well, itself, lead to attenuation of social environment and further deviance in development through perturbation of the normal genetic, social–environmental and neurodevelopmental interactions that are involved in brain growth. This has been described as a "self-perpetuating cascade"[67] of abnormal development towards schizophrenia (Figure 8).

Cognitive function and IQ before the schizophrenia syndrome

We have already noted that specific and general cognitive functions are abnormal in schizophrenia. Studies of pre-psychotic

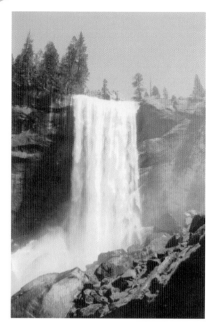

Figure 8.
Development prior to psychosis may be like a cascade, with some events and experiences early on determining the precise course thereafter, with an almost infinite number of routes to a particular place in the pool.

personality have largely confirmed the earliest clinical accounts; investigation of pre-psychotic IQ has challenged the initial notion of a deteriorating, dementing course after onset of psychosis, but the field remains controversial. Aylward *et al.*[90] have provided a comprehensive review of intelligence in schizophrenia. Standardized measures show intellectual function is lower in pre-psychotic individuals than in age-matched controls. Linking the pre-psychotic deficit to outcome, they raise the question as to whether IQ may be an independent factor that can *protect* otherwise vulnerable individuals, or whether the deficits are part of that vulnerability. Furthermore, we are not sure of what happens to this deficit over time.[91–95]

Albee *et al.*[96,97] compared childhood Stanford–Binet scores with Wecshler–Bellevue scores during adult schizophrenia psychosis in 112 people. Their longitudinal perspective allowed the authors to conclude that their results "*seriously challenge the belief that intellectual loss occurs as a consequence of adult schizophrenia*". Thirty-five years on, Russell *et al.*[98] have provided confirmatory evidence for this, but the effect remains controversial. In fact, the argument as to whether there is a developmental or degenerative process is probably a debate over a spurious dichotomy, given that a single, life-course process may be affected by a pathological process. Whether it's developmental or degenerative depends on the stage at which you begin to look at it.

In the 1946 British birth cohort (see above), several measures of educational achievement were collected on all children at ages 8, 11 and 15 years.[99, 100] The data and results are summarized by Jones[101] and show tantalizing but statistically inconclusive evidence of decline during adolescence before schizophrenia (Figures 9 and 10).

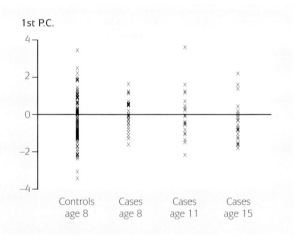

Figure 9. IQ in children in the 1946 birth cohort comparing those who did not develop schizophrenia as adults (scores at age 8 years) and those who did (scores at ages 8, 11 and 15 years). Mean scores were lower, and there was no evidence of a threshold effect below or above which this relationship did not hold. Very bright individuals did develop schizophrenia, but they were much less likely than those who are less able. Put another way, any individual is more likely to develop schizophrenia than someone who is more able in terms of IQ, although the effect is small.

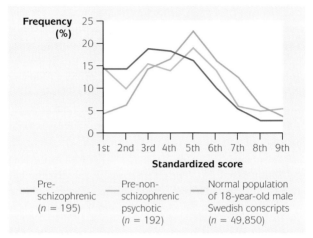

Figure 10. The same kind of relationship between pre-psychotic IQ and later schizophrenia was shown in the Swedish conscript study; here the measure was at age 18 and the left-shift consistent with a widespread effect is clear. Reproduced with permission from Cambridge University Press. David AS *et al*. IQ and risk for schizophrenia: a population-based cohort study. *Psychol Med* 1997; **27**(6): 1311–1323.[102]

Current interest in the cognitive aspects of schizophrenia[41, 57] suggests a parsimonious conclusion that pre-psychotic IQ deficits (and perhaps social characteristics) may, indeed, be manifestations of the same abnormal cognitive processes that later result in psychosis, as was suggested earlier.

The relevance of the evidence that people who develop schizophrenia may have developmental differences before psychosis begins is of relevance to clinical practice, diagnosis and prevention (Figure 11). Much more research on prediction and the specificity of these antecedent factors is required before these ideas are translated into services.[103, 104]

How many people have schizophrenia?

Prevalence data

How many people have schizophrenia at any one time? Two large studies of the prevalence of psychiatric disorders have been carried out in the US that indicate a decrease in the

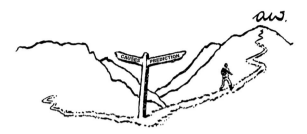

Figure 11. Much research on the developmental antecedents of schizophrenia has had the study of causes as its focus. Results that people who will develop schizophrenia have pre-psychotic abnormalities may also have relevance for clinical work and even for prevention. There is a long way to go before we can use this approach routinely. Reproduced with permission from Wainwright A. *Pictorial Guide to the Lakeland Fells. Book One; The Eastern Fells*. London: Michael Joseph.

prevalence of schizophrenia over one decade. Other major studies have been undertaken in Europe and Australia.

The Epidemiological Catchment Area programme[54] (ECA; mentioned above) surveyed 17,803 people between 1980 and 1984. This study indicated a lifetime prevalence of schizophrenia of 1.4%.[54] The National Comorbidity Survey[105] (NCS) interviewed 8098 people between 1990 and 1992 and found that lifetime prevalence for the summary category of non-affective psychosis was 0.7%.

The major prevalence study of psychiatric morbidity carried out in the UK, between April and September 1993 (OPCS), found a previous 6-month prevalence rate of only 0.4% for functional psychosis among people aged 16–64 living in private households.[106, 107] This finding was very similar to the results from a large survey of psychotic disorders embedded within the Australian National Survey of Mental Health and Wellbeing,[108] where the weighted mean point prevalence for service contact was 4.7 per 1000 adults; over 60% of these people had schizophrenia or schizoaffective disorder (http://www.health.gov.au/hsdd/mentalhe/resources/reports/pdf/overview.pdf).

While being of the same order of magnitude, there are discrepancies between these estimates from different studies; even the seemingly simple question of prevalence cannot be answered definitively. Discrepancies may be related to issues of sampling or interview methodology. They remain to be clarified by future reports. However, at present, it seems that the lifetime *prevalence* of schizophrenia in the Western world may have decreased over the past decade. This could be due to lower incidence or changes in course that would include those secondary to better treatment.

Incidence data

Changes over time

The data suggest a roller-coaster: up and down they go. It seems clear that schizophrenia became more noticeable in the population in the late 18th century and throughout the 19th (Figure 12). Whether this was due to a true increase in incidence, possibly due to new causes or greater prevalence of exposure to an old one, or to a change in the way society dealt with mental illness, is not clear. Both the late Edward

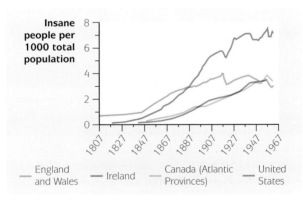

Figure 12. Counts of "insanity" rose in many parts of the West during the 19th century. Not all would have had schizophrenia, but the picture speaks for itself. Fuller Torrey E and Judy Miller. *The Invisible Plague. The Rise of Mental Illness from 1750 to the Present*, copyright ©2001 by E. Fuller Torrey and Judy Miller. Reprinted with permission of Rutgers University Press.[109]

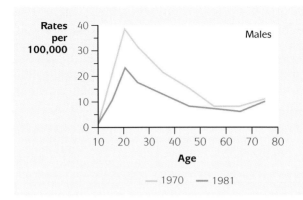

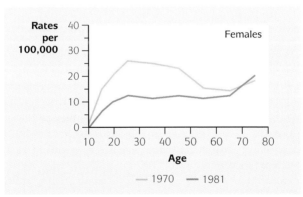

Figure 13. First admission rates for schizophrenia and paranoia by sex and age. It was shown that rates of schizophrenia seemed to have fallen in the late 20th century, but they may have gone up again. Reproduced from Der G, Gupta S, Murray RM. Is schizophrenia disappearing? *Lancet* 1990; **335**; 513–516.[110] with permission of Elsevier Science.

Hare in the UK and, more recently, E Fuller Torrey in the US[109] have written about this phenomenon extensively.

In the 20th century, the story has been one of apparent decline, then increase in a rather strange way that cannot have a single cause; the changes are dramatic (Figure 13). Eagles and Whalley[111] were first to report a decline in the diagnosis of schizophrenia among first admissions in Scotland between 1969 and 1978. Since then, there have been 14 papers examining this issue in England, Scotland, Denmark, New Zealand, Canada, Ireland, the US and the Netherlands (for a review, see Cannon and Jones[112]). In general, those based on national statistics have found a large (40–50%) decline in first admission rates for schizophrenia during the 1970s and the 1980s. However, findings based on case register data have been less consistent.

Hospital admission rates may be influenced by many factors, such as the introduction of more restrictive diagnostic criteria for schizophrenia, the move to community care, and changes in the age, sex and ethnic structure of the population. Has there really been a decrease?

Clinical experience suggests that the incidence is not decreasing, certainly not so that health services would notice. Using incidence data from a large study of first service contacts for any psychosis in Nottingham, UK and comparing these with data from a previous census that formed part of the WHO Ten Country Study,[113] Brewin *et al.* have noted an *increase* in the incidence of all psychosis categories during the 1980s and early 1990s. This was not due to an increase in any particular diagnosis, such as drug-induced psychoses. Furthermore, a third study from this city at the end of the 1990s indicates that the trend continues.

Geographical variation

The largest, multi-centre study of the incidence of schizophrenia was initiated by the World Health Organization in the late 1970s.[114] Although there was little variation between the countries for narrowly defined schizophrenia (CATEGO "S") compared with broad (CATEGO "S, P and O"), the confidence estimates for the latter estimates were wide (Figure 14). There may not have been enough power to detect considerable differences in the narrow definition,[112] and we are left not knowing whether the differences of about two-fold in broadly defined disorder are real or an artefact; the textbook point that schizophrenia occurs to a similar degree throughout the world is not really supported by even the landmark attempt to answer the question.

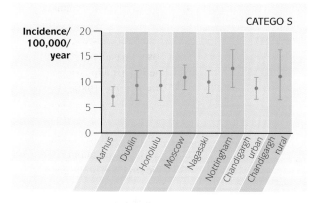

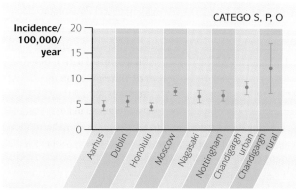

Figure 14. Incidence data from WHO Ten Country Study. Adapted with permission from Jones PB, Cannon M. Schizophrenia. In: Martyn CJ, Hughes RAC, editors. The *Epidemiology of Neurological Disorders*. London: BMJ Books, 1997.[112]

Incidence on other geographic levels – urban birth and migration

SCHIZOPHRENIA AND CITIES

The best evidence to date indicates that the incidence of schizophrenia is more common in people living in cities as compared with rural areas (Figure 15); large studies from Denmark,[115, 116] Finland,[117] the Netherlands,[118] the UK and elsewhere all show this. Moreover, it seems that the toxic period, if there is one, may be in early life.[119]

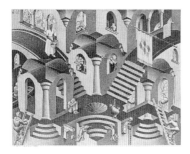

Figure 15.
Something about cities increases the risk of schizophrenia for those who live in them. M.C. Escher's 'Convex and Concave" © 2002 Cordon Art BV Baarn-Holland. All rights reserved.

This urban finding is not new. Analysis from the 1880 US census by Torrey *et al.*[120] showed this phenomenon, as did the classic study in 1920s Chicago by the social scientists, Farris and Dunham. They exploited the concentric rings of social advantage and disadvantage in that city, where the inner area is the poorest and things improve towards the suburbs (Figure 16). The figure shows that the incidence of schizophrenia estimated over 10 years is tightly related to social advantage. Causation is another matter, although drift into cities by vulnerable or ill people has been shown not to account for this, particularly given the association with early life.

The same phenomenon was found three-quarters of a century later in the city of Nottingham in the UK by Croudace *et al.*[121] (Figure 17). In this line of enquiry we are still not sure whether it is the "urbanicity", the social disadvantage or a combination of both these elusive concepts that is operating to modify risk. The phenomenon is also a good example of something clear in one research discipline (say, epidemiology) that is rather difficult to explain in another (say, psychopharmacology); that's why it's interesting! Many hypotheses have been put forward, some of the most popular being brain damage due to exposure to infectious agents and increased psychosocial stress acting as a trigger. Migration from other areas and countries may play a part, but this phenomenon, too, requires explanation.

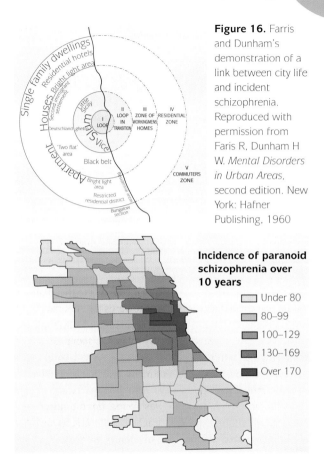

Figure 16. Farris and Dunham's demonstration of a link between city life and incident schizophrenia. Reproduced with permission from Faris R, Dunham H W. *Mental Disorders in Urban Areas*, second edition. New York: Hafner Publishing, 1960

Incidence of paranoid schizophrenia over 10 years

- Under 80
- 80–99
- 100–129
- 130–169
- Over 170

SCHIZOPHRENIA AND IMMIGRATION

Schizophrenia appears to be more common in some populations that have migrated. In 1988, the psychiatric community and beyond was surprised by a report that the incidence of schizophrenia among the African-Caribbean population in Nottingham was more than 1000% higher than in the general population.[113] Several replications from other centres in the UK[36, 122–124] and in the Netherlands[125] confirm this effect, although the true incidence ratio is now thought to be rather lower (around five-fold) when the denominator is adjusted for possible under-reporting in census data and, perhaps, due to a

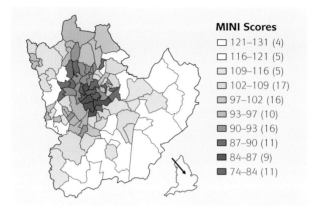

MINI Scores
- ☐ 121–131 (4)
- ☐ 116–121 (5)
- ☐ 109–116 (5)
- ☐ 102–109 (17)
- ☐ 97–102 (16)
- ☐ 93–97 (10)
- ☐ 90–93 (16)
- ☐ 87–90 (11)
- ☐ 84–87 (9)
- ☐ 74–84 (11)

Figure 17. The 2-year incidence of any psychotic illness in each electoral ward (about 4000 people) in Nottingham, UK, and the spatial association with socio-economic advantage measured with MINI, a scale summarizing a number of survey characteristics; high MINI scores indicate poorer areas. Incidence of psychosis can, effectively, be presented on the same colour scale, being most common in the deprived areas. The association between poorer areas and higher incidence of psychosis is clear, but not explained. Reproduced from Croudace *et al*.[121]

period or cohort effect.[36, 122] An increased incidence ratio for schizophrenia has also been found among African[36, 122] and Asian[122] immigrants in the UK, indicating that the effect is not confined solely to a single ethnic minority; nor, indeed is it confined to schizophrenia.[113] The hospital admission rate for schizophrenia among migrants is higher in their host country than in their country of origin,[126, 127] implicating factors occurring principally after migration. The risk of schizophrenia appears greater for second-generation migrants than first-generation migrants,[123, 124, 128, 129] arguing against selective migration of pre-schizophrenia individuals, as do the findings of Selten and Sijben.[125] The fact that immigrants from poor countries tend to show higher rates of schizophrenia than immigrants from affluent countries[130] implies that factors associated with improved living conditions, industrialization or urbanization may be involved. If we could only explain this phenomenon, we'd know a lot more about schizophrenia and its causes.

Aetiology and Diagnosis

What causes schizophrenia?

The foregoing epidemiology gives many clues to causes. It is becoming clear that most diseases are neither purely genetic nor purely environmental in origin, but depend on a complex interaction of the two.[131, 132] Twin studies are a powerful way of investigating this (Figure 18).

As the figure suggests, schizophrenia is likely to be no exception; twin studies clearly demonstrate this. Monozygotic twins share 100% of their genes, but when one monozygotic twin has schizophrenia, up to 50% of their co-twins are unaffected. Such studies clearly point to the importance of environmental factors in the aetiology of the disorder.[134] This seemingly clear logic was lost in the mid-20th century, but we are on firmer ground again now, even if we do not yet have all the answers.

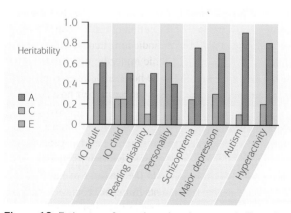

Figure 18. Estimates of genetic and environmental effects from recent twin studies. A, additive genetic variance, or heritability; C, variance from shared environment; E, variance resulting from non-shared environment and measurement errors. Data from Plomin *et al.*[133]

When we ask, "What causes schizophrenia?" Cannon and Jones[112] defined three aspects:

- What are the genes contributing to the causation of schizophrenia, where are they located, when are they expressed and for what proteins do they code?
- What environmental factors are involved in the causation of schizophrenia and when do they have their effects?
- How do the genetic and environmental factors interact with each other?

Does schizophrenia run in families?

Schizophrenia does run in families, but by no means everyone with schizophrenia has an affected relative;[135] this figure is said to be about 80% but can go down if a careful history is taken. In general, the first-degree relatives of people with schizophrenia (though this is a matter of debate of late) have a 3–7% risk for schizophrenia, five- to10-fold higher than that found in relatives of general population controls. This excess risk of schizophrenia occurs predominantly among the children and siblings of people with schizophrenia. Parents are at lowest risk; the adverse effects on fertility associated with the condition mean that parents tend to be "selected for health" and have already survived much of the period of risk (Figure 19).[136, 137]

Familiality of a disease does not necessarily imply a genetic causation. Twin and adoption studies are needed to determine to what extent the familial aggregation is due to genetic versus environmental factors.

Adoption studies

Adoption studies can tease apart the effect of family environment or styles of bringing up children from the effect of the genetic constitution of the children or parents.

The Copenhagen adoption study established a genetic basis to the familial aggregation of schizophrenia.[138, 139] The results show an increased risk of schizophrenia in the biological relatives of adoptees from parents with schizophrenia, but not in the adoptive relatives or in control adoptees. Results have been similar from a large adoption study in Finland.[140, 141]

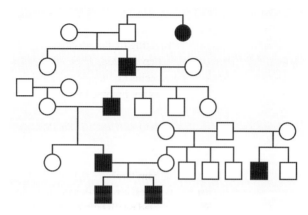

Figure 19. Schizophrenia does show familiality that is genetic, but currently there is no evidence that pushing a genetic button leads inexorably to schizophrenia; the pathway is complex.

An increased risk of schizophrenia in the absence of any contact with biological relatives indicates that genetic factors are important or necessary. Of course, this does not rule out the possibility of gene–environment interactions. Furthermore, the adopted child has still spent the prenatal period with the biological mother. However, in the Danish adoption study, the risk of schizophrenia spectrum disorders was also increased in the paternal half-siblings of the adoptee of relatives with schizophrenia that shared neither the prenatal nor the familial environment.[137]

Twin studies

Twelve major twin studies of schizophrenia have been carried out. They all show that the risk for schizophrenia in the co-twin of a schizophrenia proband (the *probandwise concordance*) is substantially higher for monozygotic (MZ; 53%) than dizygotic (DZ; 15%) twins,[135] giving an overall heritability estimate of 68% for the underlying liability to schizophrenia. Recent results from an epidemiological twin study of schizophrenia in Finland using model fitting indicates that 83% of the variance in liability to schizophrenia is due to additive genetic factors and the remaining 17% is due to unique environmental factors, with no effect for shared environment.[70] MZ discordance for schizophrenia may be caused by the "reduced penetrance" of a schizophrenia genotype, or the presence of "sporadic" or non-genetic cases. The first, but not the second, explanation would predict an increased risk of schizophrenia among the offspring of the unaffected twin of a discordant MZ pair, which has been upheld in a study by Gottesman and Bertelsen.[142] This suggests that environmental factors alone are seldom sufficient to cause schizophrenia, though they may play a decisive role in some individuals genetically predisposed to schizophrenia.

What are the genes doing?

One can think of this in two ways, in a molecular sense or in a psychological sense. Jones and Murray[143] noted that "genes code for proteins, not for delusions or hallucinations", and suggested a range of target molecules that might be involved in relevant developmental processes. Recent advances in functional genomics and proteomics are likely to take this logic forward. However, the psychological approach remains important and relevant.

Schizotypy

We have already mentioned the idea of a neuropsychological endo-phenotype, but there may also be a behavioural one that can be present without the schizophrenia syndrome. Family, twin and adoptive studies all show that certain psychiatric illnesses and personality disorders, known as the "schizophrenia spectrum", are genetically allied to schizophrenia.[144]

The most important of these disorders appears to be *schizotypal personality disorder* (SPD) (Table 13). The relative risk for SPD in the first-degree relatives of schizophrenia probands compared with controls is about five-fold.[136, 145] Parents of people with schizophrenia have a higher risk of SPD than siblings, suggesting that individuals who inherit this "milder" genetic vulnerability are responsible for the maintenance of schizophrenia in the population.[146]

Table 13. DSM-III-R diagnostic criteria for schizotypal personality disorder*

Odd communication

Inadequate rapport in face-to-face interaction

Magical thinking

Ideas of reference

Suspiciousness

Recurrent illusions

Social isolation

Undue social anxiety or hypersensitivity to criticism

Odd or eccentric behaviour

*Reprinted with permission from *Diagnostic and Statistical Manual of Mental Disorder, Fourth Edition*, Text Revision. Copyright 2000 American Psychiatric Association.

Uncertain validity and the lack of biological markers apply to SPD as much, if not more, than to schizophrenia itself. Many scales have been developed to diagnose SPD and measure "schizotypy",[147] usually self-administered questionnaires.

The major disadvantage is that the aspects of the diagnosis of SPD, which are most "predictive" of having a relative with schizophrenia, are the most subjective:[148] odd speech patterns, negative symptoms (aloofness/poor rapport), social dysfunction and avoidant symptoms, all factors that discourage participation in research. The most promising line of inquiry for diagnosis of SPD is detailed interview with *all* relatives of schizophrenia patients, particularly siblings, but this will be difficult to achieve.

The study of the siblings of people with schizophrenia is becoming increasingly popular in the field of neuropsychology.[149] Many siblings show neuropsychological abnormalities that are intermediate between the abnormalities shown by the patients and the performance of normal controls, linking these lines of psychology and personality.

"The schizophrenia spectrum"

Other disorders which form part of the "schizophrenia spectrum" are schizoaffective disorder,[137] paranoid personality disorder[146] and schizoid personality disorder,[138, 145] although there is some debate about the last of these.[146] No excess of anxiety disorder or alcoholism has been found in the relatives of schizophrenia patients compared with the relatives of controls, indicating that the genetic transmission of schizophrenia and schizophrenia spectrum disorders is relatively specific, and does not include a generalized liability to all psychiatric illness.[138, 145, 150] The debate about whether affective disorders occur to excess in the relatives of schizophrenia patients has not yet been resolved.[150–152] Relatives of schizophrenia patients do appear to have an increased predisposition to develop psychotic symptoms as part of an affective illness.[150] It may be that psychosis, or a vulnerability to it, is inherited, with other factors acting in a pathoplastic manner.

A "continuum" approach to measurement of schizophrenia

The "schizophrenia spectrum" has been talked about for many years, although little hard evidence for its existence has existed until recently. The notion of a "schizophrenia continuum" may be a more useful way to conceptualize the relationship between schizophrenia and these other disorders, particularly schizotypal personality disorder. The progression of schizotypal features into frank schizophrenia has been demonstrated,[153] though not definitively. It is also known that schizophrenia itself has a much wider range of outcome and prognoses than previously thought, with about half of patients showing "good social adjustment at follow-up" and about 20% showing almost complete recovery after one episode.[112] Few accept that a neat, categorical approach to schizophrenia is going to illuminate the truth, and some, such as Crow and Liddle, have applied different dimensional models to causation and to symptoms, respectively.

Genetic models

The true mode of inheritance is likely to be "complex".[154] Risch[155] has shown that the pattern of recurrence risks in relatives of schizophrenia probands is inconsistent with a single locus and several genome scans have now excluded this. The

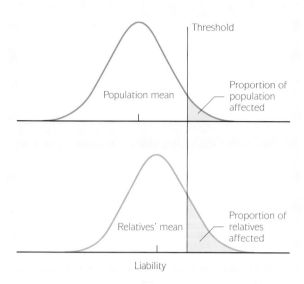

Figure 20. How the hand of genetic cards in some families means that more pass the threshold of risk or disorder than compared with the population average.

generally accepted aetiological model for schizophrenia is a combination of multiple genes and environmental factors.[144] The model has also been regarded as a liability/threshold model, with total liability above a certain value being equivalent to disease.[6, 134] On simple additive models, it is generally agreed that roughly 70% of the variation in the liability in the general population is attributable to genetic variation among individuals (Figure 20). However, this tells us little about the nature of the genetic contributions, the environmental contributions, or their interactive contributions to the risk for schizophrenia.[156]

The search for susceptibility genes for schizophrenia and quantitative traits
Genes that contribute to genetic variance in quantitative traits are known as quantitative trait loci (QTL).[157] Both linkage and

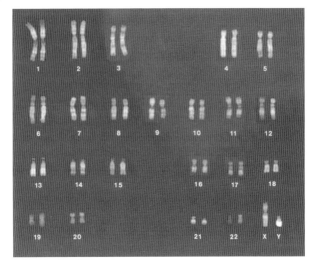

Figure 21. Genes are involved in schizophrenia but where are they and what do they do? Chromosomes 3, 6, 8 and 22 have attracted attention. Sets of functionally related genes tend to exist near to each other. Gene systems rather than individual genes may be involved, or the chance co-occurrence of otherwise neutral or even advantageous genes. Reproduced from Rimoin DL, Connor JM, Pyeritz RE, Korf B. *Emery and Rimoin's Principles and Practice of Medical Genetics, Volume 1*. Churchill Livingstone, 2001 with kind permission of Dr JR Korenberg.

association methods have been developed to map QTLs in humans (Figure 21). Another QTL approach is the use of a continuous outcome measure that is biologically related to schizophrenia, such as schizotypy.[158]

Linkage studies

Linkage analysis assesses the association of markers and alleles *within* families (Figure 22). Two common approaches are the traditional lod score approach and the more recent affected-relative-pair approach. Both have been used in the study of schizophrenia, but the latter is preferable because it does not require the mode of inheritance to be specified.[144] Further issues

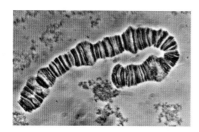

Figure 22. Linkage studies aim to show association between parts of chromosomes and characteristics or diseases so as to indicate the area of a chromosome that appears conserved or transmitted with that disease.

regarding variance and causation are reviewed by Lewontin.[159]

The Schizophrenia Linkage Collaborative Group[160] was designed to follow up on three previously published positive findings resulting from large-scale genome scans by individual groups: the 6p finding of Straub *et al.*[161] and the 3p and 8p findings of Pulver *et al.*[162] This study obtained support (but certainly not "proof") for the hypotheses that loci on chromosomes 6 and 8 have genetic variation involved in determining the level of susceptibility to schizophrenia. Fortunately, the data do seem to eliminate 3p as a candidate region. The findings for chromosome 6p generated considerable excitement.[163] It was thought at first that the susceptibility locus on 6p accounted for up to 30% of the variance in the families studied,[161] but it is now considered that only about 10% of the variance may be accounted for by this region. Another problem is that rather a large region of chromosome 6 was implicated by the positive studies, perhaps a segment containing hundreds of genes. It will be no easy task to narrow the search further.[163]

A study using a different approach – linkage to individual traits rather than to diagnosis – also implicates chromosome 6p. Arolt *et al.*[164] tested for linkage between poor eye-tracking (a phenotypic marker associated with schizophrenia) and markers on chromosome 6p in eight multiply affected families. The positive evidence for linkage was quite strong, but requires replication. Another large, international collaboration[165] was established to test positive reports of linkage between schizophrenia and an area of the long arm of chromosome 22 – D22S278. These authors concluded that if a susceptibility gene exists in this area then its contribution to the overall liability to schizophrenia is rather small, perhaps some 1%. Recent functional genomic studies have taken this further (see below).

Association studies

Association studies examine the association of disease and markers in individuals from different families.[156] For example, we could say that a population association exists between a gene and schizophrenia if those with schizophrenia were more likely than suitable controls to have a specific version of the gene.[166] A major disadvantage of association studies is that the DNA marker must be tightly linked to the disease gene. This is in contrast with the linkage method, which can detect linkage over relatively large distances.

To date, the most consistently replicated finding in this area is an allelic association between HLA-A9 and paranoid schizophrenia which has been found in seven out of nine studies.[144, 167] This association could account for about 1% of the liability to the disorder. A negative association has recently been found between schizophrenia and HLA-DR4,[168] lending support for immunological explanations for the aetiology of schizophrenia.

Anticipation

Anticipation is an inheritance pattern within a pedigree whereby disease severity increases and age of onset decreases in successive generations. This phenomenon has been described in several neuropsychiatric disorders, including fragile X, Huntington's disease and some spino-cerebellar degenerations.[169] These diseases represent a new class of disorders caused by unstable DNA sequences that can change in each generation. Such mutations depart from Mendelian inheritance, and have a highly variable phenotype with wide-ranging age at onset, both of which are well-known characteristics of schizophrenia. Anticipation has been reported in families affected with schizophrenia in two or more generations,[170, 171] and some specific trinucleotide repeats have been demonstrated in some samples.[172, 173]

The future for molecular genetic epidemiology

Linkage studies using non-parametric approaches in nuclear families and association studies using functional polymorphisms are taking over from the standard parametric lod score approach in the study of the genetics of schizophrenia.[144] As more susceptibility genes for schizophrenia are discovered there will be a move towards investigation of larger samples (usually obtained through collaboration) which are capable of detecting genes of smaller and smaller effect. Rapid and inexpensive methods of genotyping and sequencing using microchip technology are being developed and will lead to further increases in efficiency.

Functional genomics and proteomics

Technological advances in molecular biology as opposed to genetics now allow the analysis of gene expression in terms of either the amount of mRNA expressed or of proteins synthesized. These get progressively closer to the biological substrate of the purpose of genes; coding for proteins that then undergo post-translational changes and take part in biological processes. Techniques to examine mRNA and protein expression are conceptually different from molecular genetics, as well as technically distinct, because they treat genes as dynamic properties of tissues (whatever is examined), rather than fixed effects of individuals. To undertake gene expression analysis, one needs a sample of the relevant tissue, in this case the brain, so these analyses are presently undertaken on post-mortem tissue. There are prospects for analysis on peripheral tissue or cell culture. Thus, the techniques represent a new amalgam and extension of genetics, neuropathology and imaging.

Several studies have now been published, with interest aroused concerning reproducible up-regulation of several members of the apolipoprotein L family located in a high-susceptibility locus for schizophrenia on chromosome 22 (Figure 23).[174] Such findings are "causally agnostic" in that

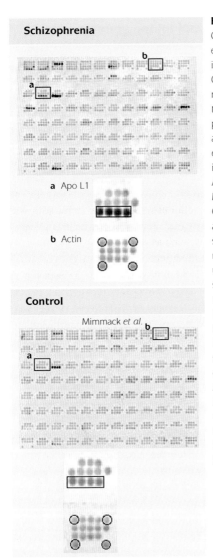

Figure 23.
Contemporary gene expression analysis in schizophrenia. Changes in regulation may themselves be primarily genetic or as a result of environmental interactions. Adapted from Mimmack ML *et al.* Gene expression analysis in schizophrenia: reproducible upregulation of several members of the apolipoprotein L family located in a high susceptibility locus for schizophrenia on chromosome 22. *Proc Natl Acad Sci USA* 2002; **99**(7): 4680–4685.[174] Copyright (2002) National Academy of Sciences, USA.

the causes of this up-regulation may be primarily genetic, environmental or due to a combination, and are not the subject of investigation. The findings may be relevant to pathophysiology though, acting through phospholipids as vital components of normal cell membranes, or as antioxidants protecting against stress triggered by infection, hypoxia or other mechanisms. Replication will confirm these techniques as crucial new tools for schizophrenia research.

Environmental risk factors

Simple additive models suggest that at least 20–30% of the variance in liability to schizophrenia may be attributable to non-genetic factors. What are these environmental factors and how might they operate? The environment can no longer be considered a "nuisance variable" by psychiatric geneticists, just as it should not be by clinicians who acknowledge the sometimes intimate relationship between their patients' experiences, their mental state and quality of life. Epidemiological clues, such as the city risk factor, serve as indicators of true risk modifiers or causes, and triggers, such as life events, are well known. What makes people vulnerable?

Many environmental risk factors appear to operate before, around or soon after birth (Table 14). Alone or together with the effects of genes, they may underpin or be manifestations of neurodevelopmental aspects of the disorder[59] that have been considered above.

Pregnancy and birth complications

People with schizophrenia, as a group, experience a greater number of labour and delivery complications than controls.[175, 176] Inspection of the particular complications associated with schizophrenia suggests that foetal hypoxia may be the common mechanism underlying these associations.[177–179]

However, labour and delivery complications, but not necessarily significant hypoxia, are relatively common in the population and are only rarely associated with schizophrenia. Other factors must play a part in a causal constellation. Taking a static approach, a particular neuronal system must be

Table 14. "Best estimate" effect sizes of various genetic and environmental risk factors for schizophrenia (expressed as odds ratios or relative risks)

Category of risk factor	Specific risk	Best estimate of effect in terms of n-fold effect
Genetic	MZ twin of someone with schizophrenia	46
	DZ twin of someone with schizophrenia	14
	Child or sibling	10
	Parent	5
Childhood developmental	Childhood CNS infection	5
	Delayed milestones	3
	Speech and language problems	3
Pre- and perinatal environment	Perinatal brain damage	7
	Rhesus incompatibility	3
	Unwanted pregnancy	2
	Severe under-nutrition (first trimester)	2
	Maternal influenza (second trimester)	2
	Season of birth (winter/spring)	1.1

damaged or extra vulnerability such as genetic predisposition must be required for schizophrenia to arise. A more dynamic, developmental view might include chance as a factor, which, along with other specific factors, determines a self-perpetuating trajectory towards psychosis,[85] as already mentioned.

Complications of pregnancy have also been associated with schizophrenia, of which the most robust are: prenatal exposure to influenza,[180–182] prenatal nutritional deprivation,[183, 184] low maternal weight,[68] rhesus incompatibility[128] and prenatal stress.[185, 186] The effect sizes associated with these prenatal risk factors are usually small (between 2 and 3), indicating that they are unlikely to be single causal agents. The association with influenza may reflect an effect related to maternal immunological responses to infection, as mentioned earlier. The association with rhesus incompatibility may be mediated through foetal hypoxia resulting from haemolysis.

Perinatal and early childhood brain damage
Recent findings from a 28-year follow-up of a Finnish birth cohort have shown that children with perinatal brain damage (defined as neonatal convulsions, low Apgar scores, asphyxia, intraventricular haemorrhage or abnormal neurological signs in the newborn period) were some seven times more likely to develop schizophrenia in adulthood than the remainder of the cohort.[73] Data from the same Finnish cohort showed that individuals who had suffered a viral CNS infection during childhood were almost five times more likely to develop schizophrenia than the comparison group.[187] The relative incidence of schizophrenia was particularly high among a group of 16 individuals who had contracted neonatal Coxackie B meningitis during an epidemic in one maternity unit. The relative effects of CNS infection are rather higher than those found for influenza in ecological studies,[152, 181] possibly due to reduction in measurement error and misclassification of viral exposure. In this study, patients with schizophrenia were also more likely to have a history of childhood epilepsy.

Foetal maldevelopment
Several studies have shown that people with schizophrenia are more likely to have had low birth weight and decreased head circumference at birth.[188] Minor physical abnormalities and dermatoglyphic abnormalities, which are thought to represent "fossilized" evidence of early developmental deviance, occur to excess in schizophrenia, as do cytoarchitectural changes, which are consistent with disturbances of development during gestation.[188] These

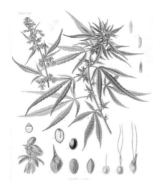

Figure 24. The cannabis plant. Picture courtesy of Royal Botanical Gardens, Kew, UK.

indicators of foetal maldevelopment may be due to a genetic process[143] or may indicate environmental insult to the foetus. A study of MZ twins discordant for schizophrenia has shown that the affected co-twin had more markers of prenatal developmental disruption than the unaffected twin.[189, 190]

Season of birth

There is a small increase in risk for schizophrenia (odds ratios (OR) of around 1.15) among individuals born in winter to early spring.[191] The reason for this "season of birth" effect is unknown,[192] although it may be a crude proxy for exposure to viral or other environmental events such as infection.

Heavy cannabis intake

Heavy cannabis consumption at the age of 18 was associated with an increased risk of later psychosis (OR 2.3) in a large cohort of military conscripts in Sweden.[193] A dose–response relationship was convincing but the direction of causality remains in question. If cannabis (Figure 24) can *cause* schizophrenia, then the apparent increase in consumption in the general population over recent decades should have led to corresponding increased rates of psychosis. As noted above, the question of trend over time is complex.

It is, however, certain that use and abuse of "street" drugs (Figure 25) is common in people with schizophrenia, and complicates management enormously. Clinical services should have very close ties with drug and alcohol services.

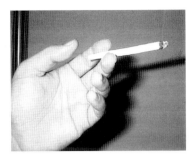

Figure 25. Cannabis use is common in people with schizophrenia, just as in people without it. Cannabis can certainly complicate treatment of schizophrenia, although initial use may ameroliate the psychological symptoms.

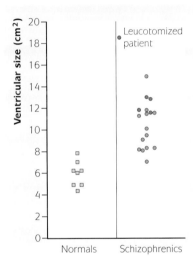

Figure 26. Ventricle : brain ratio in normal subjects and subjects with schizophrenia. This breakthrough study led people to believe all cases might be different from all controls, but this has proved not to be the case. Reproduced from Johnstone *et al*. Cerebral ventricular size and cognitive function impairment in chronic schizophrenia. *Lancet* 1976; **2**: 924–926[194] with permission from Elsevier Science.

Neither should we forget smoking tobacco, which is again very common and contributes to the excess mortality in this group.

Structural brain abnormalities and cerebral ventricular enlargement

There are small group differences between people with schizophrenia and those without (Figure 26), first identified in terms of cerebral ventricle enlargement by Johnstone *et al*.[194] over 25 years ago; their study helped put biological research in schizophrenia back on the agenda.

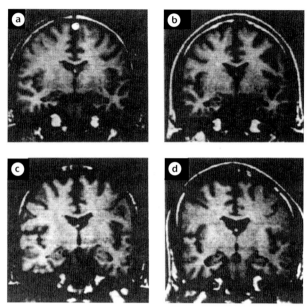

Figure 27. MRI coronal views from two sets of monozygotic twins discordant for schizophrenia showing subtle enlargement of the lateral ventricles in the affected twins (b, d) as compared with the unaffected twins (a, c), even when the affected twin had small ventricles. Reproduced with permission from Suddath RL *et al.* Anatomical abnormalities in the brains of monozygotic twins discordant for schizophrenia. *New Engl J Med* 1990; **322**: 789–794.[196] Copyright © 2002 Massachusetts Medical Society.

We don't really know if these abnormalities in cerebral structure that may underpin cognitive mechanisms of psychosis are either genetic or environmental, or more likely a combination.[195] The magnetic resonance imaging (MRI) study by Suddath *et al.*[196] of monozygotic twins discordant for schizophrenia shows that the presence of genetic risk does not account for all variance in structural differences associated with schizophrenia, and that environmental or gene-environment interactive risks are involved (Figure 27).

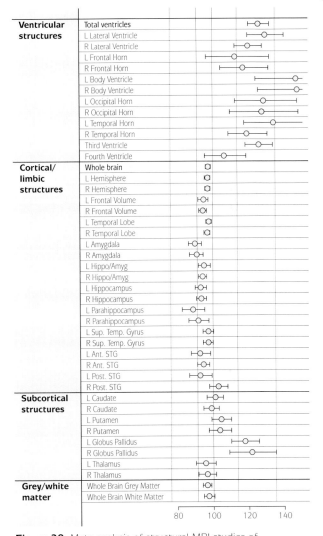

Figure 28. Meta-analysis of structural MRI studies of schizophrenia 1988–1999. Reproduced with permission from Wright I *et al.* Meta-analysis of regional brain volumes in schizophrenia. *Am J Psychiat* 2000; **157**(1): 16–25 [197] Copyright 2002, the American Psychiatric Association; http://ajp.psychiatryonline.org.

The most consistent finding is that schizophrenia patients have larger lateral ventricles than controls, with many small imaging studies yielding almost as many potential findings. A recent meta-analysis of MRI data by Wright *et al.*[197] has identified areas of consistency, and allowed the field to focus on specific areas and think about which systems may be involved (Figure 28).

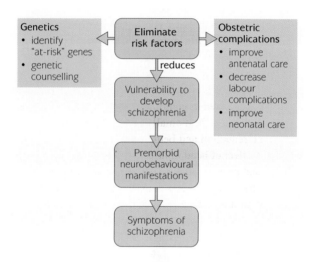

Figure 29. Prevention of schizophrenia.

Prevention

Despite substantial scientific advances over the past 15 years, the diagnosis of schizophrenia remains one of clinical judgement and the aetiological precursors for any individual patient are most often unknown. Therefore, intervening to reduce the risk of developing schizophrenia on an individual patient basis is a mammoth task.[198] Alternatively, health systems can undertake broader public health initiatives to reduce the incidence of schizophrenia.[199, 200] Improved antenatal and obstetrical care is one good example. However, there is no compelling evidence for a reduction in the incidence of schizophrenia in countries which have improved their obstetrical services over the past 20 years.[201] That does not discount an effect of improved obstetrical care, but if such an effect has occurred its contribution to the risk of developing schizophrenia is at best small. Similar prevention efforts include the reduction and better treatment of head injuries. Again, the effect of head injuries is small.

Jones and several other researchers have provided clear evidence that many patients show (in retrospect) a lifelong pattern of subtle neurological and cognitive deficits that

Stages	Possible intervention strategies
Premorbid neurobehavioural antecedents	Unknown
Prodromal stage	• Antipsychotic medications • Cognitive behavioural therapy • Psychosocial support
First episode of psychosis	• Antipsychotic medications? • Cognitive behavioural therapy? • Psychosocial support?

Figure 30. Early intervention for schizophrenia.

presage the emergence of the typical symptoms (most commonly) during adolescence or early adulthood.[74, 199] Many patients may have delayed motor milestones, neurological deficits, lower IQ than expected, attentional and related cognitive difficulties, and impairments of social and scholastic achievement. These findings, however, are non-specific and do not of themselves lead to any earlier clinical detection of schizophrenia.

Several other researchers have tried a related strategy of trying to intervene just before the onset of overt psychosis, at a time when the patient is exhibiting prodromal signs of illness but has not yet decompensated fully into psychosis.[201, 202] This approach, at least a little more focused than (earlier) intervention based on childhood biobehavioural precursors, is important because it offers the (intuitive) prospect that early intervention may prevent disease deterioration and resultant disabilities. There is some preliminary experience with the use of atypical antipsychotic medications in these at-risk groups and the results thus far are encouraging.[201–203] However, much more research is required before such an aggressive approach to medication interventions could be endorsed with confidence.

Putative approaches for preventative and early intervention models of schizophrenia management are illustrated in Figures 29 and 30.

Treatment

At present, there is no cure for schizophrenia, although, as already noted (Figure 1) there are a range of outcomes.[204, 205] Treatments are most effective when they are used in combination: pharmacotherapy, psychotherapy and social support. It is crucial that patients, family members – and also clinicians – appreciate that while we now have a range of drug treatments for schizophrenia, it is not as simple as one drug being "better" than another. Each has different indications. For example, clozapine is the drug of choice for severe schizophrenia. Each of the typical antipsychotics and the atypicals risperidone, olanzapine, quetiapine and ziprasidone (but not clozapine) are appropriate choices for early ("first-episode") schizophrenia and also for other stages of the illness.

Family involvement and support are also crucial components for success. Increasingly, as outcome improves, the need to ensure the provision of adequate vocational, housing and allied community resources will be more apparent.

The components of comprehensive disease management for schizophrenia are highlighted in Table 15.

Table 15. Comprehensive care for schizophrenia

Medication treatment

Individual supportive therapy

Cognitive and psychosocial therapies

Family psychoeducation and support

Social support

Case management

Housing

Financial support

Vocational support

Outcome of treatment has been variously defined and can be measured along many dimensions (see Figure 31). Lehman has operationalized these outcomes into proximal and distal outcomes (see Figure 32).

"Typical" and "atypical" antipsychotics – what's in a name?

Typical and atypical antipsychotic medications form the backbone of disease management for schizophrenia.[205, 206] The decision to choose a typical antipsychotic or an atypical antipsychotic medication – and which drug to use within either class – is complex. The decision should be made by the patient in collaboration with his/her doctor. Response to previous medications, sensitivity to side-effects and the pattern of the illness in that patient are all important considerations. It makes very good sense to involve family members in this decision, particularly since they may be the best judges as to how well the patient responded to previous drug treatments. It is also helpful to review any available literature to compare and

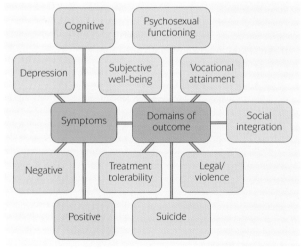

Figure 31. Multidimensional outcomes in schizophrenia.

Proximal	Distal
Positive symptoms	Functional status
Negative symptoms	Quality of life
Disorganization	Family well-being
Relational functions	Public safety
Side-effects	
Ancillary symptoms	

Figure 32. Proximal and distal outcomes in schizophrenia. From Lehman AF. Developing an outcomes-orientated approach for the treatment of schizophrenia. *J Clin Psychiat* 1999; **60**: 30–35.[204] Copyright 1999, Physicians Postgraduate Press. Reprinted with permission.

contrast each drug, so that the patient is informed as to which drug might be best for his/her circumstances. At the present time, the evidence for selecting one atypical over another is incomplete and there is still a dearth of comparative studies between these agents. Additionally, we are early on the learning curve of understanding the adverse effect profile of the atypical antipsychotics. Therefore, it is likely that practice patterns and the information accrued to determine such changes will evolve further and at a rapid pace over the next 5 years. With this in mind, it is important to understand the current distinctions between typical and atypical antipsychotic medications.

At the outset, the reader is cautioned that the current nomenclature to classify and describe antipsychotic medications is controversial and confusing.[207, 208] Older ("first generation", "conventional", "typical") antipsychotics are drugs that possess antipsychotic efficacy but are also associated with extrapyramidal side-effects (EPS). This is an essential difference between typical and atypical medications.[208] However, even here, there is a considerable "grey area" with this distinction because (i) some drugs classified as typical antipsychotics (e.g. loxapine) may (particularly when given in low dose) have a low propensity to induce EPS, and (ii) some of the atypicals (e.g. risperidone) can induce EPS, particularly if used in moderate to high doses. Also, neither

Table 16. Proposed features that differentiate atypical from typical antipsychotic medications

	Typical	Atypical
Extrapyramidal side-effects	+++	+/–
Hyperprolactinaemia	+++	+/–
Binding to mesolimbic D_2 dopamine receptors	+++	++
Efficacy for negative symptoms	+	++
Efficacy for cognitive symptoms	–	+
Effect on broader domains of outcome (e.g. depression, suicide)	+/–	+

Table 17. Classes of antipsychotic medications

Class	Example
Typical	
Butyrophenone	Haloperidol
Phenothiazine	
Aliphatic	Chlorpromazine
Piperidine	Thioridazine
Piperazine	Trifluoperazine
Thioxanthene	Fluphenthixol
Diphenylbutylpiperidine	Pimozide
Substituted benzamide	Sulpiride
Atypical	
Dibenzodiazepine	Clozapine
Benzisoxazole	Risperidone
Thienobenzodiazepine	Olanzapine
Dibenzothiazepine	Quetiapine
Benzisothiazolyl	Ziprasidone
Phenylindol	Aripiprazole
Phenylindol	Sertindole
Dibenzothiepine	Zotepine

typicals nor atypicals constitute a homogeneous group and there is wide intragroup variability (especially in adverse effect profile) between agents. Therefore, the notion that the term "atypical" appropriately describes a well-aggregated group of drugs of similar mechanism, efficacy or side-effect profile is inherently misleading. It is, however, the best working hypothesis for the present time. Other aspects which are proposed to distinguish typical from atypical antipsychotics are highlighted in Table 16.

Typical antipsychotics

The first antipsychotic medication, chlorpromazine, when originally used in anaesthesia, was noted to diminish hallucinations and delusions, and to have a calmative effect.[209] Because of these effects, antipsychotic medications were originally termed "major tranquillizers". The various classes (or subcategories) of drugs and examples of commonly used drugs are highlighted in Table 17.

Mechanism of action

Although it is unclear how these drugs work, the proposed mechanism of action of both typical and atypical antipsychotics is that they block dopamine (D_2) receptors.[210, 211] The actual scientific evidence in support of this claim comes from various sources and is summarized in Table 18. This is also illustrated in Figure 33.

These drugs also cause EPS as a direct result of their nasal ganglia.[208, 211] Recent imaging studies of the binding of drugs to D_2 receptors, as assessed using PET indicate that there is a very narrow dosing range or "window" within which one can achieve antipsychotic efficacy with typicals without causing EPS (Figures 5, 33 and 34).[212–215] Doses below this D_2 binding threshold (approximately 60% D_2 receptor occupancy) are clinically ineffective for treating schizophrenia. Doses that increase the D_2 occupancy to 70% or above will induce EPS. The atypicals, in general, have a wider therapeutic window (see later).

Table 18. Evidence for blockade of dopamine receptors as a mechanism of action of antipsychotic medications

Amphetamine, which promotes dopamine (DA) release, induces a schizophrenia-like psychosis

Antipsychotics (typicals) block DA D_2 receptors to an extent that correlates with their clinical potency

Cis-fluphenthixol isomer (which blocks D_2 receptors), but not *trans*-fluphenthixol (inert isomer), is an effective antipsychotic

Response to treatment with typical antipsychotics has been shown to correlate with changes in plasma homovanillic acid, the metabolite of dopamine

Recent PET studies confirm the need for typical antipsychotics to achieve above 60% D_2 receptor occupancy to be clinically effective

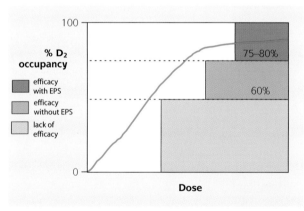

Figure 33. Dopamine receptor occupancy and clinical outcomes.

Clinical efficacy

Typical antipsychotics are effective, with an acute onset of antianxiety effect followed by a reduction in positive symptoms.[205, 216] Compared with placebo relapse rates of upwards of 80%, these drugs also reduce relapses over the course of the illness.[217] However, this advantage is lost if the

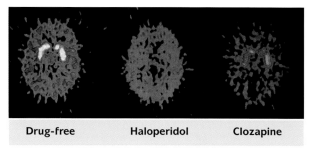

| Drug-free | Haloperidol | Clozapine |

Figure 34. Neuroimaging of antipsychotic action shows strong dopamine D_2 binding with haloperiodol but weak D_2 binding with clozapine.

dose is too low.[205] Long-acting intramuscular formulations are available and are effective options, especially when poor compliance is a concern. [218]

Unfortunately, many patients respond very poorly to these drugs.[219] Additionally, typical antipsychotics are of limited effect (and can even worsen) negative symptoms and depressive symptoms in patients with schizophrenia. They also have no appreciable effect on cognitive deficits and may even aggravate these. [220, 221]

Adverse effects

Common neurological side-effects from typical antipsychotic medications are acute dystonia, akathisia and parkinsonism.[208, 222] These effects and their management are highlighted in Table 19.

Addition of an anticholinergic drug, reduction of the dose of the typical antipsychotic or switching to a typical antipsychotic (now the preferred option) are the management choices.

Tardive dyskinesia (a more long-term effect) occurs at a rate of 5% per year for the first 5 years of treatment, with rates up to 50% in elderly populations (see Table 20).[223–225] There is evidence that clozapine reduces tardive dyskinesia and there is less but emergent data for the other agents. At

Table 19. Extrapyramidal side-effects of antipsychotic medications

Type	Mechanism	Risk factors	Treatment
Acute dystonia Oculogyric crisis and torticollis	Acute hypodopaminergia in basal ganglia	Young males, high dose, high potency, typical antipsychotics	Immediate – oral or IM anticholinergic Subsequent – reduce dose or change to atypical antipsychotic or add oral anticholinergic
Parkinsonism Bradykinesia Tremor Cog-wheel rigidity	Basal ganglia D_2 blockade	Dose related, more with typical antipsychotics	Reduce dose or add oral anticholinergic Switch to typical antipsychotic
Akathisia Motor and subjective restlessness	Basal ganglia D_2 blockade Low iron also relevant?	Low serum iron Dose related, more with typical antipsychotics	Reduce dose or add benzodiazepine/beta-blocker Switch to atypical antipsychotics

Table 20. Tardive dyskinesia	
Description	Antipsychotic-induced abnormal involuntary movements (facial, truncal, limbs)
Risk factors	Age
	Female gender
	Organic brain disease
	Prominence of negative symptoms
	Typical antipsychotic medications (predominantly) • high dose • long duration of treatment
Management	Change antipsychotic – atypical is preferred choice, clozapine has indication for treatment of tardive dyskinesia
	Other (less preferred choices) include adjunctive treatment with vitamin E or amantidine

the very least, the atypicals are far less likely to induce tardive dyskinesia (see below).

Less than 0.5% of patients exposed to treatment with typical (much less with atypicals) antipsychotics may develop neuroleptic malignant syndrome (NMS) (Figure 35).[226, 233]

Non-neurological side-effects of typical antipsychotics are highlighted in Table 21.[227]

Current indications for the use of typical antipsychotics

In America, typical antipsychotics are infrequently used and a similar but less rapid change is occurring in Europe (see Table 22). The reasons for this are varied and are enumerated in Table 22.

Pharmacoeconomic studies indicate that atypical antipsychotics are more economical than the typicals, despite their disproportionately higher prescription costs [228, 229] (because of the rapid evolution of this literature and its specificity to each country, only an overview/recent articles are provided here and the topic is not covered in detail in

Definition	Idiosyncratic patient reaction to (predominantly) typical antipsychotic medications, characterized by: • muscle rigidity • altered consciousness • pyrexia • autonomic instability • elevated creatinine phosphokinase
Risk factors	• organic brain disease • pre-existing dehydration • pre-existing agitation • rapid titration and intramuscular use of typical antipsychotic medications
Management	• stop antipsychotics • hospitalize • supportive measures – hydration, correct any electrolyte imbalance • dantrolene and/or bromocriptine may reduce morbidity of NMS episode • if another antipsychotic required, then use an atypical antipsychotic: start 2 weeks after resolution of NMS

Figure 35. Neuroleptic malignant syndrome.

this text). It appears, but is not conclusively proven by the available literature, that the atypicals are cost-effective due to less hospitalizations.

The proposed superior efficacy and enhanced tolerability of atypicals and the extent to which such attributes should dictate whether the atypicals replace the typical agents is a contentious issue, particularly in Europe. A recent article by Geddes and colleagues from England addressed this issue.[230] The authors conducted a systematic overview and meta-regression analyses of 52 randomized controlled clinical trials of the following atypical agents: amisulpiride, clozapine, risperidone, olanzapine, quetiapine and sertindole. They measured the overall symptom scores, rate of drop-

Table 21. Non-neurological side-effects of typical antipsychotic medications

Type	Treatment
Orthostatic hypotension	Lower doses, hydrate; change to antipsychotic if persistent
Hypolactinaemia • Amenorrhoea • Galactorrhoea • Complex neuro-endocrine/metabolic effects	Change to prolactin-sparing atypical antipsychotic
Sexual dysfunction • Decreased libido • Impotence • Ejaculation failure • Anorgasmia	Evaluate carefully; consider change to atypical antipsychotic
Sedation	Use less medication or less sedating antipsychotic
Anticholinergic effects • Blurred vision • Dry mouth • Constipation	Change to atypical antipsychotic
Cardiac arrhythmias • Benign • Torsade de pointes, fatal/sudden death	Increased risk with thioridazine, risk with other antipsychotics considered low
Weight gain	More common effect with atypical antipsychotics; molidone may be the least weight-inducing typical antipsychotic

Table 22. Possible reasons for the decline in use of typical antipsychotic medications in favour of atypical antipsychotics	
Pattern of use	With the introduction of atypical antipsychotics, the use of typicals has declined substantially in the USA and to a much lesser extent in European countries
Potential reasons for practice shift	Heightened marketing of atypical psychotics
	Risk of tardive dyskinesia higher with typical antipsychotics
	Superior, or at the very least comparable, efficacy of atypical over typical antipsychotics

out (~ tolerability) and side-effects (especially EPS), as recorded in these studies. They noted a substantial heterogeneity within the clinical trials, which was most readily explained by the dose of the typical antipsychotic. They reported that the evidence for superior efficacy of atypicals over typicals was weak and inconsistent between the atypicals. In addition, the authors reported that when the haloperidol dose was below/equal to 12 mg/day, atypicals proved only comparable to typical antipsychotics in efficacy and drop-out, although the new drugs still had less EPS. The authors concluded that there was insufficient evidence to support atypical antipsychotics being more effective or better tolerated than typical antipsychotics; specifically, the authors went on to recommend: "Conventional antipsychotics should be used in the initial treatment of an episode of schizophrenia unless the patient has previously not responded to these drugs or has unacceptable extrapyramidal side-effects". This article has drawn much controversy, both for and against its conclusions. Concerns have been expressed about the study's methodology, including the validity of using "drop-out" rates as a proxy to tolerability. On the other hand, it has been pointed out that the comparison between atypical and typical antipsychotic medications has become more complex over time because of the emergent side-effect profile of atypicals and that this is a (cautionary) reason for not shifting our prescribing practice overwhelmingly to the use of atypicals. Recently, another meta-analysis of randomized controlled clinical trials of atypical agents by American researchers contradicted the findings of Geddes and colleagues. Davis and colleagues conducted a meta-analysis of 100 studies for atypicals versus typicals and atypical versus atypical.[231] They found that clozapine, amisulpiride, risperidone and olanzapine were overall more efficacious than typicals; the remaining atypicals were equiefficacious with the typical antipsychotics. They also noted that the dose of haloperidol did not affect the results. They concluded that some atypicals are substantially more efficacious than typical antipsychotics, while others are not. The debate will continue. In the meantime, consumers advocate for wider availability and greater access to medications (both typical and atypical antipsychotics), citing that patients' experience of EPS is underappreciated and that the availability of choice is a major consideration.[232]

Table 23. Indications for the preferential use of typical antipsychotic medications over atypical antipsychotics	
Points of note	This is contentious, with much variability between the US and Europe in practice style
	This is in evolution
Indications	Long-term intramuscular (depot) use for poorly compliant patients
	Acute intramuscular use for agitation
	Where patient is doing well on a typical antipsychotic without evident side-effects
	When funding dictates use of less expensive drugs

At the time of writing, typical antipsychotics are appropriate for patients who are responding well and without EPS. Typicals are also used (liquid, tablet and short acting intramuscular forms) for acute agitation.[216] However, the imminent availability of short acting injectable atypicals may change this. The same is true for the current use of long acting injectable typicals. [233] Long acting atypical antipsychotics are now a new development. These current indications are highlighted in Table 23.

Atypical antipsychotic medications

Mechanism of action

Clozapine is the prototypic atypical antipsychotic medication and, in contrast to typical medications, it binds to many neurotransmitter receptors.[234] It also binds less than typical

Table 24a. Scheme of receptor antagonistic binding profile of antipsychotic medications

Drug	D_2	$5-HT_{2A}$	H_1	α_1	ACh
Haloperidol	+++	–	–/+	+	–/+
Thioridazine	+	+	+	++	++
Trifluoperazine	++	–	–/+	+/–	++
Amisulpiride	+	–	–	–	–
Clozapine	+/–	++	+++	+	++
Risperidone	+	+++	–	+	–
Olanzapine	+	++	++	+	++
Quetiapine	+/–	+/–	–	++	–
Sertindole	+	+	–	+	–
Aripiprazole*	+	++	–	–	–
Ziprasidone	+	+++	–	++	–
Zotepine	+	+	–	+	–

D_2 = dopamine D_2 receptor; $5-HT_{2A}$ = 5-hydroxytryptamine receptor, type 2A; H_1 = histamine H_1 receptor; α_1 = alpha 1 adrenoceptor; ACh = acetylcholine receptor; – = no significant receptor binding antagonism; +/– or –/+ = minimal receptor antagonism; + = receptor antagonism; ++ = moderate antagonism; +++ = strong antagonism. * displays partial agonist properties at dopamine and serotonin receptors

Table 24b. Antipsychotics safety and tolerability

Item	Typ	Clz	Ris	Olz	Qtp	Zip
EPS	+−+++	±	±−+++[a]	±−+[a]	±	±−+[a]
TD	+++	±	±−+	±(?)	±(?)	±(?)
Somnolence	±−+++	+++	±	+	++	±
Prolactin	+++	±	+++	±	±	±
Weight	±−++	+++	+	+++	+	±
Dyslipidaemia	±−+	+++	+	+++	++	±
DM	±−+	+++	+	+++	++	±
QT_c	±−+++	++	+	+	+	++
Orthostatic BP ↓	±−+++	+++	++	+	++	±

[a] = dose-related; ± = none to minimal; + = mild; ++ = moderate; +++ = marked compared to placebo rate

agents to dopamine D_2 receptors, even though it is more efficacious than typical antipsychotics. The pharmacology differs substantially between these drugs and it is at present unclear whether such differences reflect different mechanisms of action. It is also unclear whether these account for any reported differences in efficacy, adverse effect profiles or both between the currently available atypical antipsychotic medications. The relative receptor binding profiles for each of these agents is given in Table 24.

Clozapine

Clozapine was introduced in 1990 in the US and has subsequently gained wide use in the US and Europe, on the basis of the compelling findings of a carefully conducted study comparing clozapine and chlorpromazine in patients with severe ("treatment refractory") schizophrenia.[235] At the end of the 6-week trial, 30% of clozapine-treated patients were classified as treatment responders compared with 4% of the chlorpromazine-treated group (Figure 36). Subsequent studies

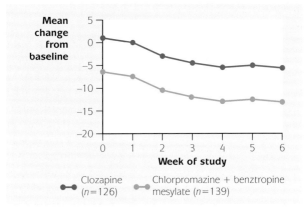

Figure 36. Clozapine versus chlorpromazine: BPRS score in treatment-resistant patients. Reproduced with permission from Kane J *et al*. The Clozapine Collaborative Group. Clozapine for the treatment-resistant schizophrenic: a double-blind comparison with chlorpromazine. *Arch Gen Psychiat* 1988; **45**: 789–796.[235]

Table 25. Use of clozapine and other atypical antipsychotic medications for specific patient subgroups

Schizophrenia

- co-morbid substance abuse
- co-morbid aggression
- tardive dyskinesia

Schizophrenia refractory to antipsychotic trials with typical (and other atypical) antipsychotics

---

and experience in clinical practice affirm clozapine's position as the treatment of choice for patients with treatment-refractory schizophrenia.[236–238] Clozapine is also indicated where patients are unable to tolerate an adequate dose of antipsychotic because of side-effects. This indication for "neuroleptic intolerance" focuses specifically on extrapyramidal side-effects and tardive dyskinesia. Clozapine has extremely low levels of EPS and, on current evidence, does not appear to cause tardive dyskinesia. In fact, clozapine is now the treatment of choice for patients with tardive dyskinesia.[239]

An important development for clozapine therapy, and for other atypical antipsychotic medications, is the understanding of its differential effects on various symptom and behavioural domains (see Figures 31, 32 and Table 25). Although the effect may lie predominantly in clozapine's low propensity to induce EPS, there is substantial evidence that negative symptoms of schizophrenia can be ameliorated, at least in part, with clozapine therapy.[240] There is also evidence that clozapine may possess thymoleptic properties and thus be beneficial in treating co-morbid mood disturbance in schizophrenia. Related to this are some important, albeit still preliminary, findings suggesting that clozapine might reduce suicidality in patients with schizophrenia.[241] There are also data to suggest that clozapine is effective in reducing persistent aggression in patients with schizophrenia.[242] Although less well studied to date, there is accruing information that clozapine may also be of particular benefit in patients with co-morbid substance abuse.[243] Finally, there is considerable evidence that clozapine can produce modest improvements in cognitive functioning in patients with schizophrenia.[220, 221] This may be a particularly important effect because of the detrimental impact of cognitive dysfunction on overall level of functioning and on the capacity for vocational rehabilitation.[244]

Clozapine is typically initiated at 25 mg per day and increased by 25 mg/50 mg per day over the first 10 days of treatment. Therapeutic doses of 300–600 mg are required. It may be necessary in maintenance therapy to titrate up to the maximum dose of 900 mg in order to obtain an adequate response. A trial of clozapine of 4–6 months duration is indicated in patients who are poor responders to other treatments.[245] Most patients respond within the first month of therapy but some may show a delayed response in the third or fourth months of therapy. It is thought that the determination of the plasma level of clozapine may be helpful to maximize efficacy.[245] Plasma levels above 400 ng/ml are recommended.

Table 26. Side-effect profile of atypical antipsychotic medications

Type	Mechanism	Risk factors	Treatment
Neurological	See Table 19: uncommon with atypical antipsychotics		
Seizures	Clozapine lowers seizure threshold	Rapid dose escalation; dose dependent – 6% at 600 mg/day	Reduce dose; add anticonvulsant
Non-neurological	See Table 21: in general, these are less common with atypical antipsychotics		
Weight gain	Complex, possibly related to antagonism of serotonin receptors	Higher baseline Body Mass Index	Dietary restriction and exercise; antiobesity agents
Diabetes mellitus	Unknown, possibly related to antagonism of serotonin receptors	Obesity; family history of diabetes mellitus	Switch to another antipsychotic medication; routine diabetic care

The main reason for the restricted use of clozapine is its side-effect profile. The side-effect profile and that of the other atypical antipsychotics is given in Table 26. The major side-effect associated with clozapine therapy is agranulocytosis.[246] This effect is seen in approximately 0.38% of patients receiving clozapine and typically occurs (80% of cases) within the first 18 weeks of therapy. This is the reason why weekly blood work is performed for the first 6 months of therapy and alternate weeks thereafter in the US. The frequency of testing in the UK is weekly for the first 6 months and then monthly; the testing frequency differs between countries. Risk factors for agranulocytosis are older age and female gender. The concomitant use of drugs known to cause agranulocystosis should be avoided – consequently carbamazepine is contraindicated with clozapine therapy. The careful monitoring of white cell counts as well as the rapid and effective use of granulocyte-stimulating factor when agranulocytosis develops have led to a negligible mortality rate with this event. Once a patient develops agranulocytosis, they must never again receive clozapine.

Seizures, generalized and myoclonic, are another serious side-effect of clozapine. Seizures occur in approximately 3–6% of patients and are dose dependent. They can be managed by reducing the dose (and going slow in titrating dose increases) and/or adding an anticonvulsant (valproic acid being the most frequent choice). A seizure is not an indication to discontinue clozapine. There have also been recent reports of clozapine-induced myocarditis and pulmonary embolism.[247, 248] These are certainly infrequent. In contrast, weight gain and metabolic disturbances are common in clozapine-treated patients.[249] Most patients gain some weight but a substantial proportion (variously estimated; conservatively 50%) of patients will become obese while on clozapine (obesity is currently defined as a Body Mass Index of 29 or greater). This may be a reason for the patient to stop taking clozapine and it is certainly a concern for the patient and the clinician regarding the long-term consequences of neuroleptic-induced weight gain. Allied to this, patients may have elevated cholesterol and plasma lipid levels; again, these are of negative long-term import.[250] More recently, it has been observed that patients receiving clozapine can show glucose intolerance (approximately 10% of patients) and some can develop overt diabetes mellitus.[251] Uncommonly, but nevertheless of great concern, some patients experience diabetic ketoacidosis. These effects are under intense research at present, both to predict which patients are at risk and to develop effective interventions.

Risperidone

Unlike clozapine, risperidone has a more targeted profile of neurotransmitter binding, with particular predeliction for dopamine and serotonin receptors.[234] Risperidone is widely used in all phases of psychosis (i.e. first episode, maintenance, treatment refractory).[252] Risperidone is best prescribed at low doses (1–4 mg/day) for the treatment of schizophrenia. Some patients may require doses of 6 mg and above, but in such instances the patient is likely to experience EPS and sometimes also sedation. Like clozapine, risperidone is effective in treating positive symptoms of schizophrenia.[253] It is also partially effective in treating negative symptoms.[254] Its efficacy to reduce co-morbid mood symptoms in patients with schizophrenia is less well established. Risperidone has also been shown in several studies to modestly improve cognitive function in patients with schizophrenia.[220, 255] There is evidence that this improvement may be most pronounced in verbal memory. There are no substantive data yet published to suggest that risperidone reduces suicidality. However, it has been shown to reduce persistent aggression in patients with schizophrenia.[256] Importantly, this drug is available in liquid form, and there are emerging data to suggest superior efficacy and tolerability of risperidone over haloperidol in the acute management of agitated psychotic patients.[216, 257]

Risperidone is used at lower doses of 1–2 mg in patients with first episode of psychosis. Emsley reported equiefficacy

(65% response rate) between risperidone and haloperidol in first-episode patients.[258] There is also evidence that risperidone is more effective than haloperidol in the maintenance treatment of schizophrenia. In a 1-year trial, there was a 23% relapse rate in patients receiving risperidone compared with a 35% relapse rate in the haloperidol-treated group.[259] There is also evidence to suggest that risperidone is effective for a proportion (perhaps 11–30%) of patients with treatment-refractory schizophrenia.

Risperidone is available in multiple tablet and also liquid form. There are also recent studies on a long-acting injectable (depot) form of risperidone.[260] This depot form has recently been approved for clinical use in several European countries and is under review in the US. The availability of a long acting form of an atypical antipsychotic (risperidone microspheres is the first but others are under development) represents a substantial advantage for the maintenance care of patients with schizophrenia, particularly for those patients with poor medication compliance.

Risperidone has a favourable side-effect profile. It has a low propensity to cause extrapyramidal side-effects, although this is dose dependent and will occur in many patients receiving doses at or above 6 mg/day. Based on current knowledge, it has a substantially lower risk of tardive dyskinesia than with typical antipsychotic medications. In a recent trial, the 1-year incidence of tardive dyskinesia was 0.6%.[259] Risperidone is associated with weight gain and diabetes, but considerably less so than most other atypical antipsychotics, particularly clozapine. Risperidone-treated patients only gained 5 lb during a recent 1-year trial. At the time of writing, risperidone is the most commonly prescribed antipsychotic in the US.

Olanzapine

Olanzapine is another atypical antipsychotic of proven efficacy.[252] It possesses a pleomorphic receptor binding pattern to neurotransmitters, with marked affinity for serotonergic and muscarinic receptors.[234] Typical doses of olanzapine for the acute and maintenance treatment of patients with schizophrenia are between 5 and 20 mg daily. The current approved upper limit for treatment is 20 mg/day, although it is not uncommon for experienced clinicians to prescribe doses above 20 mg/day for patients with treatment-refractory schizophrenia.[261]

Olanzapine has a broadly similar efficacy profile to clozapine and risperidone, in that it is effective in treating positive, negative, depressive and cognitive symptoms of schizophrenia.[262] The effects on negative symptoms are comparable to those seen with the other agents.[263] Olanzapine is effective for co-morbid mood symptoms and in fact has an approved indication in the US for the treatment of mania. In the pivotal registration trial, olanzapine was superior to haloperidol in ameliorating co-morbid depressive symptoms, with 57% of this effect being attributable to a direct effect on depression.[264] There are several studies which indicate that cognitive performance is enhanced with olanzapine therapy.[220,265]

In a recent 1-year comparative study, olanzapine proved superior to both haloperidol and risperidone on several measures of cognitive function.[265] There is at present little evidence that olanzapine reduces suicidality in patients with schizophrenia. There is strong evidence that olanzapine in a short-acting, injectable preparation is an effective and well-tolerated treatment for the acutely agitated psychotic patient.[266] There is also some early evidence that olanzapine may be an effective treatment in patients with co-morbid substance abuse.[267]

Olanzapine is an effective antipsychotic for use in first-episode schizophrenia, with typical doses being 5–10 mg. In one study, which examined efficacy in first-episode patients, 67% of olanzapine-treated patients responded compared with 29% of haloperidol-treated patients.[268] Olanzapine is also frequently prescribed as a maintenance treatment. In a study of 1 year of treatment, 14% of olanzapine-treated patients relapsed compared with 19% of haloperidol-treated patients.[269]

Olanzapine is effective in treating refractory schizophrenia.[270] Although an earlier trial of olanzapine in refractory patients proved beneficial for 7% of the olanzapine-treated group,[271] a more recent comparative trial found that olanzapine was comparable to clozapine in this patient population.[272]

Olanzapine has a favourable side-effect profile with respect to its low propensity to induce EPS or tardive dyskinesia. Extrapyramidal side-effects are not common and while there is a relationship between emergence of EPS and increasing dose of olanzapine, this relationship is much weaker than is observed with risperidone. Olanzapine has a low rate of tardive dyskinesia. In an analysis of treatment-emergent tardive dyskinesia, the incidence of tardive dyskinesia was 1.0% with olanzapine and 4.6% with haloperidol.[273] There are also early reports that olanzapine may possess an antidyskinetic effect, thus resulting in improvement in tardive dyskinesia among patients with pre-existing tardive dyskinesia.[274] Olanzapine is also less likely than either the typical antipsychotics or risperidone to induce hyperprolactinaemia.

However, olanzapine is associated with weight gain and metabolic disturbances during treatment.[247, 275] The issue of weight gain is of concern because this is a widely used drug. Many patients gain some weight but a substantial proportion (perhaps 20–30%) of patients will become obese while on olanzapine. It has been suggested that weight gain may be associated with an enhanced response to olanzapine, but this has yet to be adequately confirmed. It has also been noted that patients receiving olanzapine may develop elevated cholesterol and plasma lipid levels, and a proportion may also show glucose intolerance and/or frank diabetes mellitus.[275] These effects are less common and also less pronounced than are observed during clozapine therapy. Nevertheless, they are of concern. There is evidence that nifdizipine may reduce weight gain during olanzapine therapy.[276]

Quetiapine

Quetiapine is a dibenzothiazepine compound. It has a receptor binding profile that is broadly similar to that of clozapine.[234] Also like clozapine, studies with PET suggest that binding of quetiapine to dopamine D_2 receptors reaches a plateau (well under 50%) even when dosed up to the current maximum dose of 800 mg/day.[213] This may explain the virtual absence of EPS with this drug.[277] Kapur et al. have recently expanded this theory. They have shown that high D_2 occupancy occurs shortly after an oral dose of quetiapine, but that the drug does not persist in occupying the receptor because of its "fast dissociation constant".[278] This observation of the pharmacodynamic properties of quetiapine offers an elegant hypothesis that atypicality with these new drugs may (at least in part) be explained by a shorter period of binding to dopamine D_2 receptors. Further work is necessary to refine this hypothesis.

Quetiapine is typically prescribed at doses of 300–500 mg/day in the acute treatment of schizophrenia. Doses of 600 mg/ day and above may be required for maintenance therapy. In general, clinicians have tended to underdose this medication and they are often reluctant (despite any clear obstacle) to prescribe quetiapine at higher doses.

Quetiapine is an effective antipsychotic for treating positive, negative and overall symptoms of schizophrenia.[279] In a recent 8-week trial in patients who were partial responders to prior treatment with a typical antipsychotic, 52% of quetiapine-treated patients responded versus 38% of the haloperidol-treated patients.[280] Quetiapine's efficacy on negative symptoms is superior to typical antipsychotics and similar to that of other atypical antipsychotics. Quetiapine reduces co-morbid mood symptoms in patients with schizophrenia.[281] Quetiapine can also enhance cognitive function in patients with schizophrenia and a recent study reported superiority of quetiapine over haloperidol in several cognitive measures.[282] There is no information on the effect of quetiapine on suicidality. There are some early data to suggest that quetiapine may be helpful for patients with schizophrenia who have persistent aggression.[283] However, its effect on acutely agitated patients is less well studied and there is no liquid or acute intramuscular form available as yet.

There is less known of the role and efficacy of quetiapine as a first-line treatment for schizophrenia. However, based on the evidence for efficacy and in particular good tolerability, this drug is an appropriate choice for this patient group. Quetiapine is also an appropriate choice for maintenance therapy, although again there is less information available on this drug. There is sparse information on the use of use of quetiapine in treatment-refractory schizophrenia.[284]

Quetiapine has a particularly favourable side-effect profile. Quetiapine is essentially devoid of EPS, even at high doses. Quetiapine is also substantially less likely than typical antipsychotics to cause tardive dyskinesia, with available data showing a 1-year incidence of 0.009.[285] There is also no evidence of hyperprolactinaemia with quetiapine. There is evidence that quetiapine can cause weight gain, although this appears less pronounced than with clozapine or olanzapine.[286] There have also been reports of quetiapine-induced diabetes mellitus and cataracts. Evidence in clinical practice suggests that the drug does not cause an excess of cataracts, and post-marketing information in the US shows a lower than expected frequency of cataracts, with less opacity reported.

Ziprasidone

Ziprasidone is the most recently approved antipsychotic in the US. It is not yet available in the UK. It has a broad binding profile.[234] It is typically prescribed at doses of 80–160 mg/day, with 40 mg being the starting dose.

Ziprasidone is effective for treating positive, negative and cognitive symptoms of schizophrenia.[287] Registration clinical trials showed that ziprasidone was statistically significantly better than placebo and comparable to haloperidol in reducing psychotic symptoms.[288] There is also preliminary evidence that ziprasidone can reduce cognitive deficits in patients with schizophrenia. There is presently little information available on the efficacy of ziprasidone for co-morbid mood symptoms in schizophrenia. The effect of this drug on suicidality or on persistent aggression in patients with schizophrenia is currently unknown. However, ziprasidone is available in a short-acting intramuscular form and is an effective choice for the management of acutely agitated psychotic patients.[289]

Ziprasidone is well tolerated and has a favourable side-effect profile, especially with respect to EPS and also weight gain. Available data from clinical trials suggest that ziprasidone causes minimal EPS, even when prescribed at high doses. There is little information on the incidence of tardive dyskinesia with ziprasidone. However, there is no reason to believe that the rate of tardive dyskinesia will differ substantially from the low rates that have been observed with the other atypical antipsychotics. Ziprasidone is noteworthy for causing less weight gain than (any of) the other atypicals.[247] In a recent study in which patients were switched to ziprasidone from either typicals, risperidone or olanzapine, ziprasidone therapy was associated with a reduction in weight, particularly in patients who were previously on olanzapine.[290] Metabolic disturbances may also be less on this drug. On the other hand, concern has been raised that ziprasidone may cause cardiac conduction irregularities, specifically prolongation of the QT_c interval on ECG, in clinical practice.[291] There are data from a study which suggest that this effect may occur in a small proportion (perhaps 10%) of patients who may have QT_c prolongation above 460 ms. On the other hand, there have been no reported cases of torsade de pointes during treatment with ziprasidone and the clinical significance of any proposed cardiac effects remains to be elucidated.

Aripiprazole

Aripiprazole is the latest atypical antipsychotic to come on-line. It was available for clinical use in some European countries in late 2002 and is anticipated to be available in the US at the beginning of 2003. It has attracted considerable attention already because of its preclinical pharmacological profile (see Table 24). It is considered to be a partial agonist at dopamine D_2 receptors, that is it binds to D_2 receptors with high affinity as an agonist in the hypodopaminerigic state, while it also acts as a functional antagonist in the hyperdopaminergic state.[292–294] This apparently unique profile may confer an advantage of lower liability for EPS and hyperprolactinemia. Additionally, aripiprazole has partial agonist effects at the serotonin receptors, specifically at the $5HT_{1A}$ subtype. It is also an antagonist at the $5HT_{2A}$ receptor subtype. Collectively, it is proprosed that these effects can result in "neuromodulation" of the dopamine and serotonin systems. Therefore, the proposed mechanism of action of this drug is as a dopamine-serotonin stabilizer.[294, 295] It is important to observe, with the development of aripiprazole, how our conceptualization of the mechanisms of action of antipsychotic drugs has progressed beyond the initial idea of blocking overactive dopamine receptors.

The main information so far about aripiprazole is derived from registration clinical trials.[296–298] A placebo-controlled trial of 4 weeks duration and including over 400 patients[296] compared aripiprazole (at fixed doses of 15 mg/day and 30 mg/day) with haloperidol (10 mg/day). Aripiprazole was superior to placebo on all primary symptom measures and was equivalent to haloperidol in improving symptoms. Aripiprazole was much better tolerated in terms of EPS and prolactin elevation than haloperidol. Another placebo-controlled study trial (described in a recent meta-analysis[297]) of 4 weeks duration (within 415 patients) compared aripiprazole (at fixed doses of 20 mg/day and 30 mg/day) with risperidone (6 mg/day). Both drugs were superior to placebo on all primary symptom measures and they appeared equivalent to each other in improving symptoms. Risperidone was associated with more EPS and prolactin elevation than aripiprazole.

A recent meta-analysis of all trials conducted to date with aripiprazole confirms that this agent is efficacious for positive, negative, anxiety and depressive symptoms in patients with schizophrenia.[297] There is an absence of a dose-related increase in EPS and a favourable prolactin-sparing profile, findings that accord well with aripiprazole's proposed mechanism of action.[298] This drug also appears to be associated with a low propensity to cause weight gain, which may turn out to be a substantial advantage if confirmed in clinical practice. The cardiac profile of this drug also appears safe. Sedation appears as the most common side-effect, observed in approximately 10% of patients on 15 mg/day of aripiprazole and about 15% of patients on 30 mg/day.[298] The drug can be given as a single daily dose, with a recommendation to commence at 15 mg.

Sertindole

Sertindole is an atypical antipsychotic, a phenylindole derivative, with a high affinity as a functional antagonist at dopamine D_2 receptors, serotonin receptors (specifically the $5HT_{2A}$ receptor subtype) and α_1 adrenergic receptors (see Table 24)[299,300]. This appears, from electrochemical studies, to show a selectivity for inhibition of dopamine neurones in the ventral segmental region rather than those of the substantia nigral tract. This limbic selectivity may underlie its low liability for EPS and lack of prolactin elevation. At time of writing, it was available for clinical use in most European countries on a restricted basis for patients (who are participating in a post-marketing surveillance study) but is not presently available in the US.

The results of a major, placebo-controlled trial of sertindole (at doses of 12 mg/day, 20 mg/day and 24 mg/day) with haloperidol (4 mg/day, 8 mg/day and 16 mg/day) confirmed that sertindole is an effective antipsychotic.[301] The 20 mg/day of sertindole was the only dose of either drug to show superiority over placebo on negative symptoms. Sertindole was superior to haloperidol in terms of EPS and prolactin elevation and available information suggests that sertindole is generally well tolerated apart from retrograde ejaculation.[302] The main concern of this drug (which has also raised concern about antipsychotics as a class) has been QT_c prolongation and the risk of fatal cardiac arrhymia.[291,303] Therefore, an extensive post-marketing surveillance study is underway.[303]

The effective dose of sertindole appears to be between 12–20 mg/day, with a starting dose of 4 mg/day.

Other "atypical" antipsychotic medications

Amisulpiride and sulpiride, both from the substituted benzamide class of drugs, are widely used in Europe (especially France) in the acute and maintenance treatment of patients with schizophrenia.[304] The extent to which these drugs can be considered atypical is unclear and it appears that their neurotransmitter receptor profile is predominantly dopamine D_2 blockade. This D_2 occupancy appears to be at rates that are more in line with typical than with atypical antipsychotic medications.[234] Also, both drugs are associated with EPS and tardive dyskinesia. On the other hand, there is evidence that these drugs may have superior efficacy over typicals, and they have been shown to be superior for treating negative symptoms of schizophrenia.[305]

Zotepine is an antipsychotic, which is best considered under the group of atypical antipsychotics. It is effective for treating positive, negative and cognitive symptoms of schizophrenia.[287] Clinical trials demonstrate that zotepine is superior to haloperidol in reducing psychotic symptoms.[306] There is also some evidence that zotepine improves cognitive functioning in patients with schizophrenia. Currently, there is insufficient information on the efficacy of zotepine for co-morbid mood symptoms, suicidality or aggression in patients with schizophrenia.

Zotepine has a good side-effect profile. It has low rates of EPS and has a low incidence of tardive dyskinesia. There is insufficient information on zotepine with respect to weight gain and metabolic disturbances.

Other medications used to augment the treatment response with antipsychotics

Despite the availability of an ever-expanding range of typical and atypical antipsychotics, a substantial proportion of patients will show a partial or lack of response to antipsychotic monotherapy. Optimizing monotherapy with the chosen

Table 27. Adjunctive medications for the augmentation of antipsychotic response in schizophrenia

Drug class	Target symptoms	Preferred choice
Antipsychotics • Typical • Atypical	Positive symptoms	Typical, e.g. haloperidol
Anticonvulsants • Valproate • Carbamazepine • Lamotrigine • Topiramate • Gabapentin	Positive symptoms; agitation/ aggression	Valproate
Benzodiazepines	Agitation/anxiety	Clonezapam
Glutamatergic agents	Negative symptoms	Glycine, D-cycloserine
Anticholinesterase inhibitors	Cognitive deficits	Donezepil
Antidepressants	Depressive symptoms	Selective serotonin reuptake inhibitors

antipsychotic is the preferred strategy. Thereafter, most clinicians will choose an alternative antipsychotic as the next step in managing non-responders. However, there are several augmentation strategies that can also be tried. These include adjunctive antipsychotic medications (i.e. combining two atypicals or combining an atypical with a typical), mood stabilizers, selective serotonin reuptake inhibitors or glycinergic agents.[307, 308] These options are highlighted in Table 27. The evidence for using augmentation strategies is not compelling and this approach is associated with only modest clinical improvement. Most experts would favour switching to another antipsychotic if the observed response is

Pattern of use
• was overused in the 1960s and 1970s when diagnostic rigour between schizophrenia and mood disorder was less clear
• now infrequently used

Indications for use
• catatonic subtype of schizophrenia
• marked co-morbid depression in schizophrenia, especially with suicidality
• refractory schizophrenia, when optimized medication therapy has failed

Figure 37. Use of electroconvulsive therapy (ECT) in the treatment of schizophrenia.

Table 28. Psychotherapeutic interventions in schizophrenia		
Individual	**Group**	**Cognitive behavioural**
Supportive/ counselling	Interactive/social	Cognitive behavioural therapy (CBT)
Personal therapy		Compliance therapy
Social skills therapies		
Vocational/ rehabilitation therapies		

inadequate. Augmentation strategies are probably best restricted to the most severely ill patients who have not responded to other treatments.

Non-pharmacological management

Electroconvulsive therapy (ECT)

The role of ECT in the treatment of patients with schizophrenia is limited (see Figure 37).[309] ECT is indicated when a patient has a catatonic form of illness, a form of schizophrenia which is now considered rare. ECT is a treatment option when the patient has severe co-morbid depression. However, this is most often managed by antidepressant medications. ECT may be used when the depression is recurrent, severe and unresponsive to antidepressant treatments, and when it is associated with suicidality that is not diminished by antidepressant treatments. ECT is rarely used besides these indications of catatonia and severe co-morbid depression. It is best considered a treatment of last resort for patients with severe, refractory illness. It may be used safely with clozapine and other antipsychotic medications (see later section).

Psychotherapies (see Table 28)

There are a range of nonpharmacological, psychosocial and rehabilitative therapies, which are effective in treating persons with schizophrenia.[310, 311]

Individual

Supportive counselling/psychotherapy is an important aspect of the care of patients with schizophrenia.[312] This usually focuses on specific and daily activities, and it is not in the categories of classical or insight-oriented psychotherapy. There is ample evidence to indicate that the latter form of psychotherapy is detrimental and can result in relapse for patients with schizophrenia. However, this is often misconstrued to suggest that patients do not need or benefit from individual psychotherapy – this is simply an error. Patients need tremendous support and counselling. There are many issues that are best treated with individual psychotherapy/counselling – the meaning and impact of psychosis, insight, individual goals and life expectations, relationships with family and friends, human intimacy and sexuality, career selection, stress management, etc. Recent research has attempted to define the core elements of psychotherapy and to ascribe specific forms such as personal therapy (PT) or cognitive behavioural therapy

(CBT). PT was developed by Hogarty and colleagues at Pittsburgh, USA.[313] It views affective dysregulation and stress management as the basic focus of therapy for patients with schizophrenia. PT attempts to enhance personal awareness of each stage of illness and to promote coping skills that are appropriate to the patient's status. Hogarty et al., in a 3-year study, reported that the relapse rate with PT was lower than the alternative treatment options of either traditional supportive psychotherapy or family therapy.[313]

Cognitive behavioural therapy (CBT)
CBT in schizophrenia has been derived from its successful use in the treatment of depression.[314, 315] This therapy had been adapted for application in patients with severe schizophrenia who experience persistent and distressing delusions or hallucinations. The techniques and competencies for using CBT in patients with schizophrenia are well described. Training in CBT is important because unilateral and confrontational challenging of a patient's chronic delusional system by an unskilled clinician may place the clinician at risk of harm and may also increase the risk of relapse for the patient. There are now several studies which confirm that this is an effective treatment. One study by Sensky et al. compared CBT with "befriending therapy" in patients with chronic schizophrenia.[316] Both treatment groups showed good outcome after 6 months of treatment; however, the effect was sustained in the CBT group, who had lower symptoms and better functioning 6 months after the treatment was discontinued. This treatment has also recently been used in the care of patients with schizophrenia following their first psychotic episode.[317] The results of CBT in this less ill group are encouraging. Another development is the use of CBT to enhance the patient's adherence with treatment – so-called "compliance therapy".[318] This approach attempts to utilize the patient's level of insight and appreciation of the risks and benefits of treatment to enhance the patient's commitment and compliance with therapy. There is evidence to support a role for this modality in the maintenance therapy of patients with schizophrenia.

Family therapies

Family psychosocial therapies have arisen from the observation that patients who were stabilized on medication and then returned to families of high expressed emotion (HEE) experienced a poor outcome with relapses (see Table 29). Efforts to reduce this risk of relapse led to various psychoeducational and family therapy strategies.[310, 311, 319] Common themes that emerge in treatment with family members are listed in Figure 38. There is a large body of literature which confirms that family psychotherapy using behavioural and psychoeducational techniques can achieve superior patient outcomes compared with routine care. Relapse rates are reduced with family interventions to about 25% compared with rates of 65% among patients who receive treatment as usual.

In addition, families have formed important self-help and advocacy groups such as SANE and NAMI. It is important that clinicians recognize that family involvement is a crucial component of treatment. Also, in the wake of a voluminous literature on HEE, it is important to appreciate that family interactions are not a cause of schizophrenia.

Table 29. Stress, family involvement and medication compliance		
Patient variables		
Receiving medication	**Contact with family**	**Relapse rate 9 months post-discharge (%)**
Yes	Low expressed emotion	12
Yes	High expressed emotion, less than 35 hours contact per week	42
No	High expressed emotion, over 35 hours contact	92

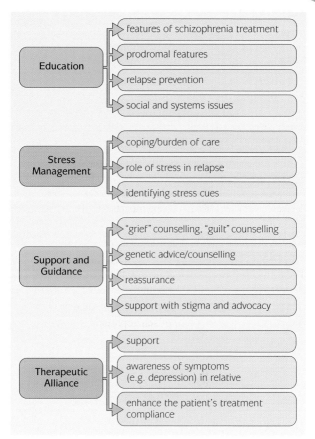

Figure 38. Themes and components of family psychotherapeutic interventions.

Social skills training

Social skills training is recognized as an important treatment modality for patients with schizophrenia.[310, 311, 320] It is based upon behavioural and learning theory techniques. Social skills therapy focuses on the discrete components of social interaction that can be identified and targeted for intervention. It is recognized that, because of the early onset of this illness, many patients will never have learnt or experienced social situations (e.g. dating) that most adults have already performed and now take for granted. Social skills training also seeks to integrate, under a rehabilitation approach, the findings of cognitive (e.g. attentional) deficits and perceptual disturbances (e.g. impaired recognition of facial emotions), that diminish the patient's capacity for normal social interactions. Three broad approaches have been identified (see Figure 39).

In the basic model, complex social repertoires are analysed and broken down into distinct steps. Each step is then role played and rehearsed until the patient has acquired the required skill. This approach has been shown to be effective, but it is not clear that these benefits tranfer into community-living situations. In the social problem-solving model, role playing is augmented with various educational activities that aim to improve the attentional and information deficits of patients with schizophrenia. Modest benefits have been demonstrated with this approach.

The observation of cognitive deficits as a core feature of schizophrenia has prompted some recent research into

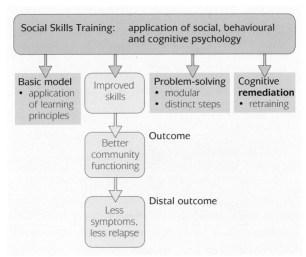

Figure 39. Social skills interventions in schizophrenia.

cognitive treatment strategies for patients.[321] One current problem is the generalizability of response from cognitive remediation training to daily situations.

Case management

Case management (CM) is the provision of supportive personnel who assist the patient in daily living and disease management.[322, 323] Allied mental health staff (e.g. community nurses, social workers or mental health "technicians") help patients to plan and attend social events, and to conduct routine tasks such as cooking, laundry and managing finances. Staff also accompany patients to outpatient visits and they will also oversee the patient's compliance with his/her prescribed medication. There are many forms of CM; generally, they vary in the intensity of service and in the patient-to-staff ratio. In the UK the Care Programme Approach (CPA) focuses on the need for a multi-dimensional care plan, regularly reviewed with the patient, and the provision of a key worker or care co-ordinator working within a multidisciplinary team. Assertive community treatment (ACT) is an important and well-studied form of CM.[322] The basic components of ACT are listed in Figure 40. This approach has been shown to reduce the hospital relapse of patients and to maintain symptom control. To achieve functional and vocational goals, it is necessary to incorporate specific social and vocational

- Outreach to patient – at home, in residential care
- 24-hour availability
- High staff : patient ratio, typically
- Frequent (daily/3–5 times per week) contact
- Co-ordinate all aspects of care – medical, psychiatric, social
- Functional performance and satisfaction (patient, family) are more important outcomes than symptom reduction

Figure 40. ACT programme characteristics.

strategies into the overall treatment plan. There has been considerable research in an effort to determine which is the most appropriate and most effective CM model for patients and what type of personnel (e.g. nurses or technicians) are best suited to provide this from of "home care". In general, the service types are equivalent in outcome, and show improvements in rehospitalization rates and overall quality of life. However, they have been less effective in getting patients back to work, which most consumers would consider an essential outcome measure.

Vocational rehabilitation

Vocational rehabilitation is a critical but most often underresourced component of the comprehensive care of patients with schizophrenia. Only about 20% of patients achieve any form of employment and more often than not this is either sheltered employment or low-skilled and poorly paid work. Sheltered workshop and supportive work therapies have been shown to increase the quality of life and to sustain employment in patients.[324] However, rates of relapse remain high in these patients and unfortunately it is often only the least symptomatic patient who can withstand the stress of regular work without relapse. Recently, Bell *et al*. showed that a neurocognitive enhancement therapy added to work produced substantial improvements in cognitive function among patients with chronic schizophrenia.[325]

Systems issues

Despite substantial treatment advances, we often provide care in mental health systems that is inadequately funded, poorly planned and often executed in a disjointed fashion. The optimal treatment for schizophrenia is not always used in clinical practice. There are often discontinuities between inpatient and outpatient care. Additionally, there is wide variability in the clinical practice. Patients may receive different medications based on the prescribing practices of psychiatrists rather than any clear distinctions in illness. There is sometimes disjointed care where, in spite of the availability and support for use of atypical antipsychotics, medications are switched too frequently and patients are exposed to periods of no treatment. In addition, there is considerable variability in the extent and quality of psychosocial and vocational services that are available to patients. There is also concern as to the "fidelity" of the practiced model of service. For example, many services would claim to provide ACT, but when these services are evaluated with respect to the key elements of the ACT model they are found to fall short. Future directions in health services research and delivery will be to integrate social skills and assertive CM interventions with other approaches, such as vocational training, housing support, etc. The challenge to integrate our services is immense. Making real progress in treating schizophrenia requires attention to these many other needs, as well as providing availability to new medications. Integrating these components and tailoring these to the needs of the individual patients is the real challenge of comprehensive and continuous care for schizophrenia.

Management

Acute psychosis

The goals of acute management are:

- To conduct a careful assessment of symptoms and behaviour of psychosis
- To evaluate and provide immediate management of the risk of suicide, if any exists
- To evaluate and provide immediate management of the risk of harm to others, if this risk exists
- To institute immediate measures to stabilize psychosis and to plan further care

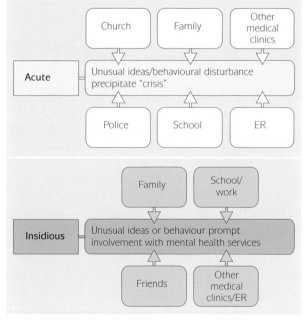

Figure 41. "Pathways to care" for patients with first-episode psychosis.

Figure 42. Other causes of first-episode psychosis which can resemble schizophrenia.

- Organic brain disorders
  - head trauma
  - epilepsy
  - sarcoidosis
  - infections (HIV, encephalitis)
  - vasculitis (SLE)
  - multiple sclerosis

- Drug-induced psychotic disorder

- Brief psychotic disorder

- Mood disorder with psychosis

- Delusional disorder

The acutely psychotic patient often presents in crisis (see Figure 41).

It is essential to conduct a thorough assessment in order to arrive at a presumptive or definitive diagnosis and also to plan for immediate care. Ruling out other conditions is an important first step of management (see Figure 42). As outlined earlier, a wide variety of general medical and central nervous system conditions can present with psychotic features that mimic schizophrenia. Additionally, psychotic symptoms related to substance abuse are often difficult to distinguish from schizophrenia. This circumstance may be further complicated by co-morbid substance abuse in patients who have a diagnosis of schizophrenia. Also, psychotic symptoms associated with schizophrenia may be similar to those seen in schizophreniform disorder, brief psychotic disorder, delusional disorder, schizoaffective disorder or bipolar disorder. Determining the correct diagnosis(es) is essential to treatment planning. Core aspects of the assessment of the acutely psychotic patient are highlighted in Table 30. The evaluation of risk of self-harm and harm to others is of particular importance. Alongside how florid the patient's psychosis is, these are the main reasons why a patient will be admitted to hospital as opposed to being cared for in a day hospital or in another outpatient setting.

Table 30. Assessment of the patient presenting with a first psychotic episode

Historical	Onset and duration of illness
• Rule out other aetiologies	Antecedent factors – head injury
• Confirm diagnosis	Substance abuse Medical history History from relative/ close friend
Observational	Level of consciousness
• Rule out other aetiologies	Symptoms of psychosis
• Confirm diagnosis	Presence of mood features
• Evaluate treatment needs	Neurological evaluation Level of agitation
Ancillary	Laboratory tests
• Rule out other aetiologies	• Haematology
• Confirm diagnosis	• Metabolic
• Support treatment planning	• Drug and alcohol
	Neuroimaging
	Detailed collateral information, including assessment of carers' needs

The use of medications in the acutely psychotic patient are highlighted in Table 31. Acutely psychotic patients who are agitated will require immediate pharmacotherapy.[216] Every effort should be made to acquire informed consent to treatment from the patient. If medications are necessary and the patient consents, then medication treatment should be given in oral tablet or liquid form. Unfortunately, it is not uncommon for patients who present as acutely psychotic to deny their illness and, consequently, refuse medication (and often all other forms) of treatment. At this juncture, the clinician is at an impasse and he/she must carefully weigh the immediacy and extent of risk against the competency and expressed wishes of the patient. When the risk of harm is imminent and serious, immediate action is required and the patient should be

Table 31. Choice of medication interventions in the acutely psychotic patient

Option	Management
Antipsychotic	Low dose to minimize potential for side-effects; use more sedating drug if agitation is a problem; use acute intramuscular preparation if risk to self/others
Benzodiazepine	Use – not routine; use if agitation; use intramuscular preparation if agitation is a substantial problem
Chloral hydrate	Use – not routine; use if agitation or insomnia

involuntarily medicated. In this (unfortunate) circumstance, medication must be given in intramuscular form. The most frequently used medications by intramuscular route are typical antipsychotics and/or a short-acting benzodiazepine. It is likely that atypical antipsychotics will be used more in this circumstance once they become available in short-acting intramuscular form.

If the risk of harm is serious but less immediate – and the patient still refuses treatment – then the clinician must decide whether to commit the patient to hospital against his/her will.[326] The procedures and legal requirements for involuntary commitment differ substantially from country to country.

If the risk of harm is low but the patient is in need of continued observation because of the degree of psychosis, then the clinician must decide whether hospitalization or day treatment is appropriate. This will depend on many factors, chief of which are the extent of the patient's psychosis (especially the amount of behavioural control and insight the patient exhibits) and the extent of support the patient has.

First-episode psychosis

Patients may present acutely, with florid psychotic symptoms, or they may come to treatment after a long and insidious onset of illness; the latter is associated with poorer treatment response and poor long-term outcome. The importance of a thorough assessment at the beginning of treatment cannot be emphasized enough. Although clinicians differ on the extent of medical evaluation at the onset of psychosis, most would consider it prudent to order some routine biochemical and imaging tests (see Tables 4, 5 and 30).

There is no clear choice of any particular antipsychotic as the first-line treatment. In Europe, clinicians often commence therapy using one of the typical antipsychotics, although this practice is changing rapidly. In the US, clinicians now almost invariably prescribe an atypical antipsychotic as the first-line treatment. As is the case with the typicals, there is no guidance (as of yet) as to which of the atypical agents is the best option. It is likely that the atypical agents are essentially equiefficacious in this highly responsive population and at present there are no direct comparative studies published to inform clinical practice.

Studies of risperidone and olanzapine in first-episode schizophrenia have been described in an earlier section. It is important to appreciate that patients experiencing their first episode of psychosis are at a stage of illness that is, in general, more responsive than later to medication and other treatments.[327] They are also much more sensitive to the adverse effects of medications. For both reasons, clinicians usually begin treatment with low doses of the chosen antipsychotic medication. In the acute, hospital setting, the medication may be increased every 2–3 days depending on tolerance and response. With this approach, one can expect to reach an appropriate maintenance dose in a matter of days.

On the other hand, if the patient is less psychotic and is being treated as an outpatient, then the escalation of dose will be slower and will occur typically over the course of several weeks. In either instance, it is critical that the patient and clinician be alert for the emergence of side-effects. Failure to recognize and effectively treat adverse effects in first-episode patients leads to non-compliance with therapy; this will ultimately result in a relapse of psychosis. The adage "start low and go slow" is useful when initiating antipsychotic therapy in this group.

Table 32. Themes and components of counselling for the first episode of psychosis	
Education	Features of schizophrenia
	Treatment options
	Prodromal features and relapse prevention
	Social support and information on resources, disability support, with focus on recovery.
	Tackling drug misuse
Role clarification and outcome expectations	"Grief" counselling
	Clarification of likely short-term, intermediate treatment outcomes
	Functional, social, occupational goal setting
	Reintegration

It is also critical to provide supportive psychotherapy/counselling during (and after) this first episode of psychosis. Aspects that are the focus of therapy at this stage are highlighted in Table 32. CBT has also been shown to be an effective treatment at this stage of the illness.[317]

Maintenance therapy

Effective maintenance treatment can decrease the frequency and the severity of the episodes of illness, reduce its morbidity and mortality, and maximize the psychosocial functioning and the quality of life of patients. While some patients have an excellent outcome and therefore only need periodic monitoring, most patients require comprehensive and continuous care over the course of their illness.

With regard to medication treatments, the benefit of maintenance pharmacotherapy must be balanced against the risk of long-term side-effects of treatment.[205] The positive impact of typical antipsychotic medications on the course of illness has been highlighted earlier. These drugs reduce relapse and can improve functioning. Their main drawback in long-term therapy is the risk of tardive dyskinesia. This risk can be minimized by using the lowest effective dose of the typical antipsychotic medication (see earlier section). There is insufficient information on the longer-term efficacy and in particular comparative trials of atypical antipsychotics. The favourable results of the 1-year relapse prevention study of risperidone versus haloperidol[259] were described earlier. There are also direct comparative trials of risperidone versus olanzapine, and risperidone versus quetiapine. In a 28-week double-blind study, patients receiving risperidone and patients receiving olanzapine improved over time.[328] There was evidence for superiority of olanzapine over risperidone with respect to the amelioration of depressive and negative symptoms. The olanzapine-treated patients also had generally fewer side-effects. However, not unexpectedly, the olanzapine-treated patients experienced more weight gain (4.1 ± 5.9 kg versus 2.3 ± 4.8 kg). This study was conducted shortly after both risperidone and olanzapine became available in clinical practice and the dosing profiles (mean modal doses: olanzapine, 17.2 ± 3.6 mg/day; risperidone, 7.2 ± 2.7 mg/day) are unbalanced, particularly the dose of risperidone, which is in excess of current dosing in clinical practice. In a smaller and more naturalistic 6-month follow-up study[329] of patients being treated with either risperidone (6 mg/day) or olanzapine (14 mg/day), both drugs proved comparable in efficacy during the first 4 weeks of acute treatment, but risperidone proved superior for overall amelioration of psychotic symptoms at 6 months. Another 8-week, double-blind prospective trial compared risperidone (mean modal dose of 4.8 mg/day) with olanzapine (12.4 mg/day) in patients with chronic schizophrenia.[330] Risperidone-treated patients showed a greater improvement in positive and anxiety/depression symptoms. Rates of EPS were comparable between both drugs. More weight gain occurred in the olanzapine group. There is also information on the comparative efficacy of risperidone and quetiapine, based upon a 4-month open-label trial[281] of quetiapine (mean dose 254 mg/day) versus risperidone (mean dose 4.4 mg/day) in patients with psychotic disorders (almost

75% of patients had a diagnosis of either schizophrenia or schizoaffective disorder). Both drugs were efficacious across a range of symptoms, with a slight advantage for quetiapine in treating depressive symptoms. Quetiapine was also associated with less EPS.

In the absence of convincing and substantial comparative trials of each atypical antipsychotic in refractory schizophrenia, choice of medication in this patient group is, in part, being influenced by their relative adverse effect profile. The adverse effect profile of antipsychotic medications is a major issue in the maintenance treatment of schizophrenia. It is argued that atypical antipsychotics are better tolerated than typicals and that this is a major justification for favouring atypicals for long-term management. In one recent study,[331] side-effects, subjective tolerability and impact on quality of life were compared between patients receiving typical antipsychotics ($n = 44$) and those receiving atypicals (risperidone, $n = 50$; olanzapine, $n = 48$; quetiapine, $n = 42$; clozapine, $n = 46$). Patients receiving atypical antipsychotics experienced fewer side-effects overall (especially EPS and neuroleptic-induced dysphoria), more positive subjective responses and favourable attitudes to treatment; no significant difference emerged on any of these measures between each of the atypicals. On the other hand, there is now substantial concern that atypicals induce weight gain and metabolic disturbances, which may have serious long-term health consequences.[249, 332] In a 5-year report of 101 patients who had been treated with clozapine for at least 1 year,[250] weight gain was maximal during the first year of treatment, but patients continued to gain weight up to month 46. Of considerable concern is the high rate (52% at the end of 5 years) of new-onset diabetes mellitus. There was a non-significant increase in total serum cholesterol and a significant increase in triglycerides. In another study[275] of weight gain and metabolic disturbance in patients treated, on average, for 6 months with olanzapine (median dose of 12.5 mg/day), 57% of patients had a body mass index above normal, 20% had hyperglycaemia, 71% had elevated insulin levels, 62% hypertriglyceridaemia,

85% hypercholestrolaemia and 57% had elevated leptin levels. In the maintenance therapy of schizophrenia, we are currently evaluating when and how best to screen patients and implement treatment strategies for weight gain, diabetes mellitus and other metabolic disturbances.

The impact of concern over cardiac effects of antipsychotic medications in the management of (treatment-refractory) schizophrenia is another issue in the long-term management of schizophrenia. The reader is referred to two recent comprehensive reviews of cardiotoxicity of antipsychotic medications, in particular QT_c prolongation and the risk of torsades de pointes.[291,333] Another analysis of outpatients at a British centre found that QT_c prolongation was associated with the use of either thioridazine, droperidol or high-dose antipsychotic therapy.[334] There have also been recent reports of fatal myocarditis–cardiomyopathy and pulmonary embolism during clozapine therapy.[247, 248] It is now considered prudent to obtain an ECG at regular intervals (perhaps annually) in patients on maintenance pharmacotherapy with antipsychotic medications.

Several key points can be made about the maintenance pharmacotherapy of schizophrenia. First, treatment response remains highly individualized and although there is ample evidence that each of the antipsychotics described above is effective in treating schizophrenia, it is difficult in an individual patient to predict whether one drug or another will prove effective. It is hoped that the new research direction of pharmacogenetics may in time provide better predictive ability.[335] Second, while there is emerging evidence for class superiority of atypical over typical antipsychotic medications in the maintenance therapy of schizophrenia, there are as yet too few data to distinguish with any confidence treatment differences between each of the atypical agents. Where differences emerge, it is typically with respect to the side-effect profile of these drugs. Third, it is exceedingly common (in approximately 30% of patients in the US) for patients to be treated with various combinations of medications – either a typical antipsychotic with an atypical, two atypicals together, an antipsychotic plus a mood stabilizer, an antipsychotic plus a benzodiazepine, or

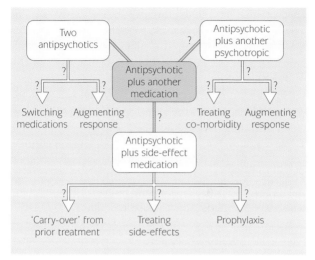

Figure 43. Rational polypharmacy in schizophrenia.

Table 33. Switching from one antipsychotic to another

Risks	Somatic withdrawal symptoms
	Relapse of psychosis
Management	Avoid "cold turkey"
	Cross-taper
	• gradual phase-out of first medication
	• gradual increase of new medification
	Avoid leaving the patient "stranded" on two drugs

any combination thereof (Figure 43).[336, 337] The merits of this practice and the optimum choice of polypharmacy are presently unknown. Fourth, because we have had a spate of new antipsychotics in recent years, we are still very much in a learning phase with respect to the optimum dosing and duration of clinical trial of each drug. Therefore, there is wide variability in clinical practice with respect to how long a trial and at what dose of agent a patient will be treated with before changing to another drug. Inevitably, this gap in knowledge and the variability in treatment leads to frequent switching between these drugs.[338] This itself is a major issue. Guidelines for switching from one drug to another are given in Table 33.

The focus of psychological support during maintenance therapy needs to be broad and also individualized to the patient's needs. Issues of relevance to counselling may range from acquiring friendship, interviewing for part-time employment, to human sexuality.[312] The clinician needs to possess the same skills and empathy for the patient's dilemmas as he/she might for any other patient that is more "high functioning". CBT may help to reduce delusions and hallucinations, although this modality is best practised by a skilled clinician.[315] This approach may also be used to enhance the patient's long-term compliance with therapy, so-called "compliance therapy".[318]

Treatment-refractory schizophrenia

Despite optimum care, a substantial proportion of patients (perhaps 30%) will fail to show an adequate response to treatments.[270] These patients with treatment-refractory (TR) schizophrenia constitute the most difficult to treat group. They are also the patients who are disproportionate users of the mental health (emergency and legal) services.

Clozapine is the treatment of choice for TR schizophrenia. This is confirmed in several studies and key meta-analyses (see "Prevention" section). As yet, there is insufficient information on the comparative efficacy of clozapine and the other atypical antipsychotics. Available studies are conflicting and difficult to interpret, in part because of variable definitions of treatment resistance. On balance, these currently point to clozapine's advantage in severe TR schizophrenia. On the other hand, they also show that some TR patients will respond to other atypical antipsychotics (see Table 34).

Information on the use of other atypical antipsychotic medications is emerging. For risperidone, there is evidence that this drug is effective in a proportion of refractory patients.[339] For olanzapine, Breier *et al*. have analysed data on

Table 34. Pharmacotherapy of "treatment-refractory schizophrenia"	
Agent	**Efficacy**
Typical antipsychotics	"By definition" ineffective
Clozapine	Effective in possibly 60% of patients
Risperidone	Effective, but less so than clozapine
Olanzapine	Effective, probably less so than clozapine, although some data show comparability
Quetiapine	Efficacy at high doses, but extent is undetermined at present
Ziprasidone	Undetermined at present
Aripriprazole	Undetermined at present
Sertindole	Undetermined at present
Zotepine	Undetermined at present

patients with treatment-refractory schizophrenia ($n = 526$) who were a subgroup of the multicentre comparative trial of olanzapine versus haloperidol.[340] In a last observation carried forward analysis, olanzapine-treated patients showed greater response rates than haloperidol-treated patients (46% versus 35%). On the other hand, Sanders and Mossman found that only two of 16 patients with severe schizophrenia/schizoaffective disorder showed a significant response to olanzapine.[261]

Which medication (i.e. which drug in what order, and when) sequence is the best is still very unclear. Available treatment guidelines do not distinguish one atypical from another. On current evidence, there seems to be no defined rationale for starting with one drug instead of the other. Also, which drug to try next is unclear, and at present this choice is largely driven by patient preference and an appreciation of the relevant side-effect profile of each drug. At what time point the clinician should resort to clozapine therapy is also unclear. Clozapine is underutilized in the US and Europe, in part because clinicians have relegated it to the treatment of last resort, after trials of several of the atypical antipsychotics. In one study of refractory patients with prior exposure and inadequate response to risperidone, haloperidol and then olanzapine, 50% of patients then responded to a trial of clozapine.[341] This observation is important because it confirms the clinical impression that failure to respond to one atypical antipsychotic does not preclude response to another agent. However, we still lack clear guidance as to the appropriate sequence (and dose) of trial of each agent and when, if warranted, to proceed to clozapine therapy.

What to do when clozapine therapy fails is a real dilemma.[308] One approach is to try adding in several agents to augment the response to clozapine (see Figure 44). These approaches are more of a trial-and-error. In one recent study, glycine, an N-methyl-D-aspartate (NMDA) receptor agonist, was added to clozapine therapy in 27 patients with schizophrenia.[342] There was no observed benefit to adding glycine, in contrast to the beneficial effect of NMDA agonists in augmenting response to typical antipsychotic medications.

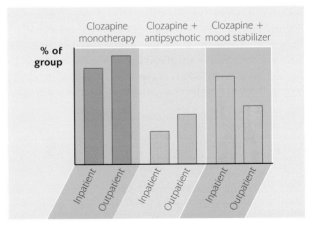

Figure 44. Co-pharmacy with clozapine. Reproduced from Buckley PF et al. When symptoms persist: clozapine augmentation strategies. *Schizophrenia Bull* 2001; **27**: 615–628.[308]

ECT is another treatment option for patients with refractory schizophrenia who have failed other treatment options. A recent literature review of ECT augmentation of clozapine response suggests that 67% of patients benefit from augmentation with ECT. Adverse effects (prolonged seizures, non-fatal cardiac arrhythmias) occurred in 17% of patients.[309] ECT should only be considered for treatment-refractory patients following a careful review of prior treatments and after a second opinion has been obtained from another psychiatrist.

There are now several studies demonstrating the efficacy of CBT for persistent delusions and hallucinations (see Table 35).[311, 314, 315] In one study, refractory patients received CBT or supportive counselling. Both groups improved during the 9 months of therapy. However, the CBT group continued to improve beyond the treatment period.[316] CBT is a useful modality but its cost effectiveness needs to be determined. ACT is another important intervention.[323]

Co-morbidities
Depression and suicide
Depression is common in patients with schizophrenia.[343] At least 50% of patients become depressed at some stage during their illness. Depression is associated with more frequent relapses and with a poorer outcome. Depression in schizophrenia is also associated with suicide. It is critical for mental health professionals to appreciate this close association and to be of heightened awareness of the risk of suicide in

Table 35. A randomized, controlled trial of cognitive behavioural therapy for persistent symptoms in schizophrenia resistant to medication

CBT has been shown to be useful in schizophrenia

Patients in the study received 9 months on CBT or non-specific befriending while receiving medication and case management

Both groups improved over 9 months, but the CBT kept improving for the 9-month follow-up patients with schizophrenia who exhibit signs of co-morbid depression.[344] It is reliably estimated that approximately 50% of patients attempt suicide at some point during their illness. Awareness of the factors that may contribute to suicide among people with schizophrenia and the early detention of and intervention with people who are at risk for suicide are key components for successful management. There is also emerging information suggesting a positive impact of present day pharmacotherapy on suicidality in schizophrenia.[345] The main element of this work concerns the atypical antipsychotic clozapine and several studies show that, through some yet to be elucidated mechanism, clozapine appears to exert an antisuicidal effect in people with schizophrenia.[346] Potential mechanisms for this putative antisuicidal effect may include a (direct) thymoleptic effect, an enhancement of insight (either directly and/or indirectly through improved cognition), or enhanced quality of life on this medication such that the patient is not overwhelmed by the hopelessness of intractable illness. An antisuicidal effect of clozapine (and perhaps other atypical antipsychotics) is an intriguing proposition and is consistent with heightened treatment expectations that extend beyond amelioration of symptoms to ultimately more profound domains of outcome in schizophrenia, specifically suicide and aggression.

Violence

Although rates vary widely depending upon the population studied and the definition of violence, approximately 15% of patients with schizophrenia exhibit violent behaviour.[347] Active psychosis is a prominent risk factor for violent behaviour in schizophrenic patients and, although there are some associations between particular symptom constellations (the "threat–control override" pattern), the evidence for distinct symptoms as risk factors is less pronounced than one might intuitively consider. Substance abuse is also a major risk factor for the occurrence of violence in schizophrenic patients. Non-compliance with medication, inextricably linked with an active co-morbid substance and with psychotic decompensation, is another prominent risk factor.[348] A prior history of aggressive behaviour and of being abused as a child are other risk factors. At the same time, however, since risk factors such as substance abuse, acute psychotic decompensation and command hallucinations are all too common features in the course of schizophrenia, it is hardly surprising that these are, at best, only modest gauges of the imminent risk of violence – arguably the strongest clinical predictor. The prediction of imminent risk of violence is heightened by the closer the temporal relationship to prior violence, the presence of signs of acute agitation and actual threats of violence. The pharmacological management of the acutely agitated/aggressive patient has been covered earlier.

The pharmacological management of persistent aggression in patients with schizophrenia is complex. Because such patients are often non-compliant with treatment, they are appropriate candidates for a trial of a long-acting intramuscular antipsychotic. However, their illness is frequently unresponsive to standard treatments and these patients often receive multiple medication combinations. These combinations are changed frequently on a trial-and-error basis. There is emerging evidence that clozapine may be a particularly effective treatment for schizophrenic patients with persistent aggression. Beyond medication, the management of their care is more complex because it brings social and legal issues to the fore. The management of the patient with schizophrenia who has a history of violence constitutes a careful balance between the patient's clinical/personal needs and the perceived risk of violence for the community at large, i.e. societal needs. Since control of illness is a key principle of managing the risk of violence, then contentious treatment options, such as forced medication or involuntary hospitalization, must be considered.[349] These approaches are, to a large extent, logical from a clinical perspective of risk management – particularly given the accruing evidence that risk of violence is interrelated with level of disease activity – but they juxtapose serious ethical and social concerns that already have a long and inglorious history in the care of people with serious mental illness.

Co-morbid substance abuse

Substance abuse co-morbidity (SA) in schizophrenia is a major concern, both in view of the frequency of SA among patients with schizophrenia and the notorious difficulty in managing such patients. The ECA study reported a prevalence of SA at 47% among patients with schizophrenia.[350] The consequences of SA in schizophrenia are extreme. These patients are much greater users of psychiatric services. In addition, they are seen more frequently by the emergency services and are more likely to use jail services. Available evidence suggests that the long-term course of SA in patients with schizophrenia is poor, both in terms of the persistence of SA and the poor outcome in substance-abusing patients. Elements of comprehensive care are outlined in Table 36. Treatment programmes emphasize many of the 12-step approaches that are advocated in the treatment of primary alcoholism and SA. In addition, they emphasize the development of social skills, behavioural management and motivational enhancement therapy.[351] The pharmacological management of co-morbid SA in schizophrenia is less well studied. There are emerging clinical data to suggest that atypical antipsychotics, particularly clozapine, may be beneficial in the management of patients with co-morbid substance abuse and schizophrenia.[352]

Co-morbid obsessive-compulsive symptoms with schizophrenia

Obsessive-compulsive symptoms, co-morbid with schizophrenia, occur in approximately 5–7% of patients.[353] Although the presence of obsessive-compulsive disorder (OCD) symptoms was though to predict a better outcome, these feature typically characterize a poor outcome and intractable symptoms. It is unclear as to how to treat these symptoms and there is evidence that these features can uncommonly emerge *de novo* during treatment with an atypical antipsychotic medication. Selective serotonin reuptake inhibitors have been tried but their use is complicated by their effect of elevating the plasma level of the antipsychotic. Given

Table 36. Comprehensive care for people with schizophrenia

1. Best practices pharmacotherapy

Is dynamic

Reflects current literature

Is consistent with established standards of care

Needs to be integrated with other services/supports

Can synergize with other modalities

2. Responsibilities of the clinician in prescribing antipsychotic medications

Clinicians need to discuss:

- risks and benefits
- side-effects

Should have leaflets and educational handouts available

3. Setting goals for medication treatment

Specific

Measurable

Consistent with standards of care

Consistent with established outcome expectations

"Stable on current medications" may be too low an expectation of treatment outcome

4. Establishment of a strong continuum of care for best practices pharmacotherapy

Clinicians need time, support and resources to communicate effectively with other clinicians. These resources include:

- clear documentation of medications
- appropriate sharing of documentation and prescription details
- clinician-to-clinician discussion of medication treatments

such a pharmacokinetic interaction, these drugs should be used with caution during clozapine therapy.

Future Developments

The pace of new drug development for schizophrenia is exciting and offers hope to patients and their relatives. Several drugs are at advanced stages of development. These new drugs represent refinements of current proposed mechanisms of drug action and/or new mechanisms (Figure 45). For example, iloperidone, currently at the advanced stage of clinical drug development, is a drug that has a similar receptor binding profile to clozapine. It has been shown in early studies to be an effective antipsychotic.[354]

There is also interest in examining the role of sigma receptor antagonists, GABA agonists and other highly selective agents in the treatment of schizophrenia. There is also substantial interest in the role of antioxidants in the treatment of schizophrenia, this work being based upon the findings of phospholipid abnormalities in patients with schizophrenia.[355] At present, these approaches are experimental and are not recommended for clinical practice.

Neural system	Focus/effect
Dopamine receptors	Partial agonist – antagonism Highly selective antagonist
Serotonin receptors	Highly selective antagonist (with or without dopamine antagonism)
Sigma receptors	Antagonist
Glutamate receptors	Agonist/antagonist
CNS phospholipid metabolism	Omega-3 fatty acid supplements
CNS oestrogen receptors	Oestrogen

Figure 45. New mechanisms of action of putative novel antipsychotics/antipsychotics under development.

There is also interest in the role of pharmacogenetics to enhance the prediction of patient response to antipsychotic medications.[335] In one recent study,[356] six polymorphisms of serotonin receptor genes were highly predictive (with a sensitivity of 95%) of a response to clozapine. This focus of research has substantial potential and clear relevance for the management of schizophrenia and it raises the (currently far-off) possibility that we may in the future be able to individualize treatment regimes.

There is also a more general trend in the US toward greater integration of mental health and medical care for people with schizophrenia.[357] It is increasingly being recognized that patients with schizophrenia have high rates of physical co-morbiditity and that this clinical dilemma may be further complicated by the medical effects (obesity, diabetes mellitus, cardiotoxicity) of the atypical antipsychotic medications. Consequently, there is an emerging trend towards greater involvement of other medical specialists in the care of people with schizophrenia. In the UK, the move to integrate mental health and social care may mitigate against this.

There is also evidence that the management of schizophrenia will be increasingly influenced by the evidence-based medicine (EBM) approach.[358, 359] This will be of assistance in providing the context for appropriate pharmacotherapy, as well as ensuring that health care systems provide the full range of services (ACT, case management, vocational support) that are of proven effectiveness in the long-term care of people with schizophrenia (Figure 46).

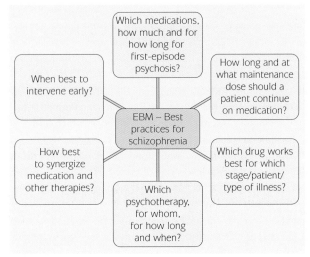

Figure 46. Evidence-based medicine (EBM) and schizophrenia.

Frequently Asked Questions

Is there a test for schizophrenia and can it be used to "diagnose" family members at risk?

Unfortunately, there is no test that can readily diagnose schizophrenia. The diagnosis is still essentially based on the clinical presentation and exclusion of other medical conditions that can mimic schizophrenia. There are several abnormalities (e.g. eye-tracking deviations) that are seen in patients and also in their families. However, these are not of diagnostic value and at present are of no clinical value in determining whether an asymptomatic family member will develop schizophrenia.

Does drug abuse cause schizophrenia?

People with schizophrenia often abuse drugs and it is not uncommon to encounter the situation where patients have abused drugs prior to their illness. One is then left wondering "would he/she have developed schizophrenia if he/she had not abused drugs?" There is some evidence that cannabis use may induce schizophrenia in some patients. There is less known about other drugs. In general, however, it is (far) more likely that the drug use is part of the patient's coping response to the onset of psychosis or simply a co-occurrence (epiphenomenon) rather than being the cause. Also, drug-induced psychoses tend to be brief in duration and do not last like schizophrenia.

How violent are people with schizophrenia?

The public perception and understanding of schizophrenia is that most patients are likely to be violent and that patients have a "Jekyll and Hyde" predisposition for violence. This is grossly overestimated, although perhaps some 10% of patients exhibit violent behaviour. Violence typically occurs during periods of relapse and is most often associated with alcohol/drug use and non-compliance with medication treatment. Most violence is of low lethality, although some patients can be very dangerous and in need of long-term institutional care to minimize the risk to society.

If the illness is caught early can it be treated with a better outcome?

This is a major question for our field at the present time. It may be possible to identify people who are in the prodromal phase of their illness and intervene early to reduce their long-term morbidity. This is intuitive. However, it is not proven and it is possible that earlier treatment may just forestall the onset of illness and not really impact the course of illness. However, much like other chronic medical illnesses, we believe that intervening early will lead to a better outcome. Proving that is the real challenge. See Section 1 for further discussion.

How long should a person continue on medication?

This is a difficult question to be dogmatic about and certainly the answer "for the rest of your life" does not sit well with patients or their families. If somebody is in their first episode of schizophrenia and has completely remitted signs of illness, then it is reasonable to consider gradually reducing medication after 1 year of treatment. This is about the most optimistic circumstances and unfortunately most patients do end up on medication indefinitely.

How do you choose "the right medication" and how do you know it is "the right one"?

At present, there is no way of guiding clinicians as to which drug will be optimum for which patient. Also, there is a large overlap with respect to efficacy between each of the typical antipsychotic medications and also between each of the atypical antipsychotics. Side-effects distinguish better between all of these drugs. Therefore, it is somewhat a process of trial and error to find the drug that works best and has the fewest side-effects for any given patient. There are some broad approaches – e.g. use a more sedating medication for an agitated patient, avoid an antipsychotic with high risk of weight gain in an obese patient.

How long should you wait on one drug before switching to another drug?

This depends on several factors, particularly the extent of response and the extent of side-effects that the patient is experiencing on his/her present medication. Usually, it is recommended that a patient receive a 6–8 week trial of an antipsychotic. This may need to be longer if the dose of medication was too low. On the other hand, the trial might be appropriately aborted before 8 weeks if the patient experiences distressing or serious side-effects. It is generally considered that a longer trial period (probably about 4 months) is required to adequately assess a patient's response to clozapine.

What is the best combination of medication treatments?

In general, antipsychotic monotherapy is preferred and should be the practice until it has failed or there is an emergence of other co-morbid side-effects that do not respond to this treatment. There is no obvious or "best" choice of medication combination. The choice is usually guided by the target symptom – i.e. another antipsychotic for persistent positive symptoms, an antidepressant or mood stabilizer for co-morbid affective symptoms or a selective serotonin reuptake inhibitor for co-morbid obsessional symptoms.

Are other treatments, such as herbals, helpful in the treatment of schizophrenia?

There is little or no evidence that herbal and alternative medicine treatments have any meaningful role to play in the treatment of schizophrenia. There is, however, some evidence that "fish oil" may be a beneficial supplement to augment the response of antipsychotic medications; fish oil is not, however, considered a primary treatment for schizophrenia. There is also some preliminary evidence that hormonal therapy with oestrogen may enhance the response to antipsychotic medications.

How do you "convince" a person with schizophrenia to comply with their medication treatment?

This is a huge problem and there are no good answers yet. It is important to try and understand why it is a patient will not take their medication – e.g. it may be that they are experiencing a distressing side-effect that could be alleviated. There is also now a form of CBT called "compliance therapy" that targets the circumstances of poor compliance. So far, results of studies using compliance therapy are encouraging.

If somebody suspects schizophrenia, who should you contact to get help for them?

There are a range of options, depending on the severity of illness and the acuity of the presentation. Obviously, somebody who is psychotic and says he/she is going to kill himself and/or somebody else needs to be evaluated immediately. In this case, bringing the person directly to the emergency department is an appropriate response. Somebody who has shown subtle signs of gradual deterioration over time might be more appropriately scheduled for an outpatient consultation with a psychiatrist. Other ways to get help – and to access mental health services – include contacting the family physician, contacting a mental health professional such as a psychologist or counsellor, or contacting a support/advocacy organization such as NAMI or SANE.

References

1. Andreasen NC. Symptoms, signs and diagnosis of schizophrenia. *Lancet* 1995; **346**: 477–481.

2. Susser MW. *Causal Thinking in the Health Sciences. Concepts and strategies in epidemiology.* New York: OUP, 1973.

3. Murray RM, Lewis SW, Reveley AM. Towards an aetiological classification of schizophrenia. *Lancet* 1985; **i**: 1023–1026.

4. Kendell RE. Schizophrenia: the remedy for diagnostic confusion. *Br J Hosp Med* 1972; **8**: 383–390.

5. Clare A. *Psychiatry in Dissent: Controversial Issues in Thought and Practice.* Tavistock, UK, 1979.

6. Zubin J, Spring B. Vulnerability – a new view of schizophrenia. *J Abnorm Psychol* 1977; **86**(2): 103–126.

7. American Psychiatric Association. *Diagnostic and Statistical Manual of Mental Disorders*, 4th edn. Washington, DC: American Psychiatric Association, 1994.

8. World Health Organization. *The ICD-10 Classification of Mental and Behavioural Disorders: Diagnostic Criteria for Research.* Geneva: World Health Organization, 1993.

9. International Early Psychosis Association: http://www.iepa.org.au/.

10. McGorry PD. The recognition and optimal management of early psychosis: an evidence-based reform. *World Psychiat* 2002; **1**(2): 76–83.

11. Shepherd M, Watt D, Falloon I, Smeeton N. The natural history of schizophrenia: a five year follow up and prediction in a representative sample of schizophrenics. *Psychol Med.* Monograph Suppl 1989; **15**: 1–46.

12. Lewis SW. The secondary schizophrenias. In: Hirsch SR, Weinberger DR, editors. *Schizophrenia.* Cambridge: Blackwell Science, 1995; pp. 324–340.

13. Ron M, Harvey I. The brain in schizophrenia. *J Neurol Neurosurg Psychiat* 1990; **53**: 725–726.

14. Guze SB. Biological psychiatry: is there any other kind? *Psychol Med* 1989; **19**: 315–323.

15. Bynum WF. Psychiatry in its historical context. In: Shepherd M, Zangwill OL, editors. *Handbook of Psychiatry*, Vol. 1. Cambridge: CUP General Psychopathology, 1983; pp. 12–13.

16. Murray RM. Neurodevelopmental schizophrenia: the rediscovery of dementia praecox. *Br J Psychiat* 1994; **165**(Suppl 25): 6–12.

17. Kraepelin E. Dementia praecox. In: *Psychiatrie*, 5th edn. Leipzig: Barth, 1896; pp 426–441. Translated in: Cutting J, Shepherd M. *The Clinical Roots of the Schizophrenia Concept.* Cambridge: CUP, 1987; pp. 13–24.

18. Kraepelin E. Dementia praecox and paraphrenia. Translated by Barclay RM from: Robertson G, editor. *Text Book of Psychiatry*, Vol. iii, Part ii, section on Endogenous Dementias, 8th edn. Edinburgh: Livingstone, 1919.

19. Pick A. *Über Primäre Demenz*. Wandervorträge, 1891.

20. Diem O. Die einfach demente Form de Dementia praecox. *Arch Psychiat* 1903; **37**: 111–187.

21. Pinel Ph. *Traité Médico-philosophique sur l'Aliénation Mentale*. Paris: R. Caille, Ravier, 1801.

22. Morel BA. *Etudes Cliniques: Traité Théorique et Pratique des Maladies Mentales*. Paris: Masson, 1852.

23. Morel BA. *Traité des Maladies Mentales*. Paris: Masson, 1860.

24. Snell L. Uber Monomanie als primäre Form der Seelenstörung. *Allg Z Psychiat* 1865; **22**: 368–381.

25. Kahlbaum KL. *Die Katatonie oder das Spannungsirresein*. Berlin: Hirschwald, 1874.

26. Hecker E. Die Hebephrenie. *Virchows Arch Pathol Anat* 1871; **52**: 394–429.

27. Fink E. Beitrag zur Kenntnis des Jugendirreseins. *Allg Z Psychiat* 1881; **37**: 490–520.

28. Bleuler E. Die Prognose der Dementia Praecox – Schizophreniegruppe. *Allg Z Psychiat* 1908; **65**: 436–464. Translated in: Cutting J, Shepherd M. *The Clinical Roots of the Schizophrenia Concept*. Cambridge: CUP, 1987; pp. 59–74.

29. Bleuler E. *Dementia Praecox oder Gruppe der Schizophrenien*. Leipzig, Vienna: Deuticke, 1911.

30. Murray RM. Schizophrenia. In: Hill P, Murray RM, Thorley A, editors. *Essentials of Postgraduate Psychiatry*. Cambridge: CUP, 1986; pp. 339–379.

31. Minkowski E. Le trouble essential de la schizophrenie *et al*., pensee schizophrenique. *La Schizophrenie*, Chap. 2. Paris: Payot, 1927. Translated in: Cutting J, Shepherd M. *The Clinical Roots of the Schizophrenia Concept*. Cambridge: CUP, 1987; pp. 189–212.

32. Stransky E. Towards an understanding of certain symptoms of dementia praecox. Zur Auffassung gewisser Symptome der Dementia Praecox. *Neurol Centralblatt* 1904; **23**: 1137–1143. Translated in: Cutting J, Shepherd M. *The Clinical Roots of the Schizophrenia Concept*. Cambridge: CUP, 1987; pp. 36–41.

33. Castle DJ, Murray RM. The neurodevelopmental basis of sex differences in schizophrenia. *Psychol Med* 1991; **21**: 565–575.

34. Schneider K. *Clinical Psychopathology*. Translated by Hamilton MW. New York: Grune & Stratton, 1959.

35. Cooper JE, Kendell RE, Gurland BJ *et al. Psychiatric Diagnosis in New York and London*. Oxford: Oxford University Press, 1972.

36. van Os J, Castle DJ, Takei N, Der G, Murray RM. Psychotic illness in ethnic

minorities: clarification from the 1991 census. *Psychol Med* 1996; **26(1)**: 203–208.

37. Jackson JH. *Selected Writings of JH Jackson*. London: Hodder & Stoughton, 1931.

38. Crow TJ. Positive and negative symptoms of schizophrenia and the role of dopamine. *Br J Psychiat* 1980; **137**: 383–386.

39. Andreasen NC. *Can Schizophrenia be Localised in the Brain?* Washington, DC: American Psychiatric Press, 1986.

40. Carpenter WT Jr, Heinrichs WD, Alphs LD. Treatment of negative symptoms. *Schizophrenia Bull* 1985; **11**: 440–452.

41. David AS, Cutting J. *The Neuropsychology of Schizophrenia*. Hove: Lawrence Erlbaum, 1994.

42. Braff DL. Information processing and attention dysfunctions in schizophrenia. *Schizophrenia Bull* 1993; **19**: 233–259.

43. Mesulam MD, Geschwind N. On the possible role of the limbic cortex and its limbic connections in the process of attention in schizophrenia. *J Psychiat Res* 1983; **14**: 249–261.

44. Ingvar DH, Franzen G. Abnormalities of cerebral blood flow distribution in patients with chronic schizophrenia. *Acta Psychiat Scand* 1974; **50**: 425–462.

45. Liddle PF, Friston KJ, Herold S *et al*. A PET study of word generation in schizophrenia. *Schizophrenia Res* 1994; **11**: 168.

46. Wernike C. *Grundrisse der Psychiatrie*. Leipzig: Thieme, 1906.

47. Jones PB. The early origins of schizophrenia. *Br Med Bull* 1997; **53**(1): 135–155.

48. Lewis SW. Congenital risk factors for schizophrenia. *Psychol Med* 1989; **19**: 5–13.

49. Murray RM, Jones PB, O'Callaghan E, Takei N, Sham PC. Genes, viruses and neurodevelopmental schizophrenia. *J Psychiat Res* 1992; **26**(4): 225–235.

50. Kostovic I, Rakic P. Developmental history of the transient subplate zone in the visual and somatosensory cortex of the macaque monkey and human brain. *J Comp Neurol* 1990; **297**(3): 441–470.

51. McGuire PK, Frith CD. Disordered functional connectivity in schizophrenia. *Psychol Med* 1996; **26**: 663–667.

52. Friston KJ. Dysfunctional connectivity in schizophrenia. *World Psychiat* 2002; **1**(2): 66–71.

53. Hirsch SR, Shepherd M. *Themes and Variations in European Psychiatry*. Bristol: John Wright, 1974.

54. Keith SJ, Regier DA, Rae DS. Schizophrenic disorders. In: Robins LN, Regier DA, editors. *Psychiatric Disorders in America: the Epidemiologic Catchment Area Study*. New York: Free Press, 1991; Chap. 3.

55. Eaton WW. Update on the epidemiology of schizophrenia. *Epidemiol Rev* 1991; **13**: 320–328.

56. Heaton RK, Baade LE, Johnson KL. Neuropsychological test results associated with psychaitric disorders in adults. *Psychol Bull* 1978; **85**: 141–162.

57. Green MF. What are the functional consequences of neurocognitive deficits in schizophrenia? *Am J Psychiat* 1996; **153**: 3.

58. Häfner H, Riecher-Rossler A, An Der Heiden W *et al*. Generating and testing a causal explanation of the gender difference in age at first onset of schizophrenia. *Psychol Med* 1993; **23**(4): 925–940.

59. Weinberger DR. Schizophrenia: from neuropathology to neurodevelopment. *Lancet* 1995; **346**: 552–557.

60. Erlenmeyer-Kimling L, Cornblatt B, Friedman D *et al*. Neurological, electro-physiological and attentional deviations in children at risk of schizophrenia. In: Henn FA, Nasrallah HA, editors. *Schizophrenia as a Brain Disease*. New York: OUP, 1982; pp. 61–98.

61. Fish B. Infants at risk for schizophrenia: sequelae of a genetic neurointegrative defect. *Arch Gen Psychiat* 1992; **49**: 221–235.

62. Fish B. Neurobiological antecedents of schizophrenia in children. *Arch Gen Psychiat* 1977; **34**: 1297–1313.

63. Walker E, Lewine RJ. Prediction of adult-onset schizophrenia from childhood home movies of the patients. *Am J Psychiat* 1994; **147**: 1052–1056.

64. Marcus J, Hans SL, Auerbach JG *et al*. Children at risk for schizophrenia: the Jerusalem infant development study. *Arch Gen Psychiat* 1993; **50**: 797–809.

65. Wadsworth MEJ. Follow-up of the first national birth cohort: findings from the Medical Research Council National Survey of Health and Development. *Paediat Perinatal Epidemiol* 1987; **1**: 95–117.

66. Wadsworth MEJ. *The Imprint of Time. Childhood History and Adult Life*. Oxford: Clarendon Press, 1991.

67. Jones PB, Harvey I, Lewis SW *et al*. Cerebral ventricle dimensions as risk factors for schizophrenia and affective psychosis: an epidemiological approach to analysis. *Psychol Med* 1994; **24**: 995–1011.

68. Crow TJ, Done DJ, Sacker A. Childhood precursors of psychosis as clues to its evolutionary origins. *Eur Arch Psychiat Clin Neurosci* 1995; **245**: 61–69.

69. Done DJ, Johnstone EC, Frith CD *et al*. Complications of pregnancy and delivery in relation to psychosis in adult life: data from the British perinatal mortality survey sample. *BMJ* 1991; **302**: 1576–1580.

70. Cannon TD, Kaprio J, Lonnqvist J *et al*. The genetic epidemiology of schizophrenia in a Finnish twin cohort: a population-based modelling study. *Arch Gen Psychiat* 1998; **55**(1): 67–74.

71. Jones P, Rodgers B, Murray R, Marmot M. Child development risk factors for adult schizophrenia in the British 1946 birth cohort. *Lancet* 1994; **334**:1398–1402.

72. Rantakallio P. Groups at risk in low birth weight infants and perinatal mortality. *Acta Paediat Scand Suppl* 1969; **193**: 1–71.

73. Isohanni M, Jones PB, Moilanen K *et al*. Early developmental milestones in adult schizophrenia and other psychoses. A 31-year follow-up of the North Finland 1966 birth cohort. *Schizophrenia Res* 2001; **52**: 1–19.

74. Poulton R, Caspi A, Moffett TE *et al*. Children's self reported psychotic symptoms and adult schizophreniform disorder: a 15 year longitudinal study. l. *Arch Gen Psychiat* 2000; **57**: 1053–1058.

75. Cannon M, Caspi A, Moffitt T *et al*. Evidence for early, pan-developmental impairment specific to schizophreniform disorder. Results from a longitudinal birth cohort. *Arch Gen Psychiat* 2001; **59**(5): 449–456.

76. Gervin M, Browne S, Lane A *et al*. Spontaneous abnormal involuntary movements in first episode schizophrenia and schizophreniform disorder: baseline rate in a group of patients from an Irish catchment area. *Am J Psychiat* 1998; **155**: 1202–1206.

77. Ambelas A. Preschizophrenics: adding to the evidence, sharpening the focus. *Br J Psychiat* 1992; **160**: 401–404.

78. Cannon-Spoor HE, Potkin SG, Wyatt RJ. Measurement of premorbid adjustment in chronic schizophrenia. *Schizophrenia Bull* 1982; **8**(3): 470–484.

79. Foerster A, Lewis SW, Owen MJ, Murray RM. Pre-morbid adjustment and personality in psychosis. Effects of sex and diagnosis. *Br J Psychiat* 1991; **158**: 171–176.

80. Gittleman-Klein R, Klein DF. Premorbid and social adjustment and prognosis in schizophrenia. *J Psychiat Res* 1969; **7**: 35–53.

81. Robins LN. *Deviant Children Grown Up. A Sociological and Psychiatric Study of Sociopathic Personality*. Baltimore: Williams & Wilkins, 1966.

82. Watt N, Lubensky A. Childhood roots of schizophrenia. *J Consult Clin Psychol* 1976; **44**: 363–375.

83. Watt NF. Patterns of childhood social development in adult schizophrenics. *Arch Gen Psychiat* 1978; **35**: 160–165.

84. Done DJ, Crow TJ, Johnstone EC, Sacker A. Childhood antecedents of schizophrenia and affective illness: social adjustment at ages 7 and 11. *BMJ* 1994; **309**: 699–703.

85. Jones P, Rodgers B, Murray R *et al*. Childhood developmental risk factors for schizophrenia in the 1946 national birth cohort. *Lancet* 1994; **344**: 1398–1402.

86. Malmberg A, Lewis G, David A, Allebeck P. Premorbid adjustment and personality in people with schizophrenia. *Br J Psychiat* 1998; **172**: 308–313.

87. Reichenberg A, Rabinowitz J, Weiser M *et al*. Premorbid functioning in a national population of male twins discordant for psychoses. *Am J Psychiat* 2000: **157**: 1514–1516.

88. Rabinowitz J, Reichenberg A, Weiser M *et al*. Cognitive and behavioural functioning in men with schizophrenia both before and shortly before first

admission to hospital. Cross-sectional analyses. *Br J Psychiat* 2000; **177**: 26–32.

89. Cannon TD, Rosso IM, Hollister JM *et al.* A prospective cohort study of genetic and perinatal influences in the etiology of schizophrenia. *Schizophrenia Bull* 2000; **26**(2): 351–366.

90. Aylward E, Walker E, Bettes B. Intelligence in schizophrenia: meta-analysis of the research. *Schizophrenia Bull* 1984; **10**: 430–459.

91. Hunt JMcV, Cofer C. Psychological deficit. In: Hunt JMcV, editor. *Personality and the Behavior Disorders*. New York: Ronald Press, 1944.

92. Hunt H. A practical clinical test for organic brain damage. *J Appl Psychol* 1943; **27**: 275–286.

93. Lubin A, Gieseking CF, Williams HL. Direct measurement of cognitive deficit in schizophrenia. *J Consult Psychol* 1962; **26**: 139–143.

94. Mason C. Pre-illness intelligence of mental hospital patients. *J Consult Psychol* 1956; **20**: 297–300.

95. Rappoport SR, Webb WB. An attempt to study intellectual deterioration by pre-morbid testing. *J Consult Psychol* 1950; **14**: 95–98.

96. Lane EA, Albee GW. Childhood intellectual development of adult schizophrenics. *J Abnorm Soc Psychol* 1963; **67**: 186–189.

97. Albee GW, Lane EA, Corcoran C, Werneke A. Childhood and inter-current intellectual performance of adult schizophrenics. *J Consult Psychol* 1963; **27**(4): 364–366.

98. Russell AJ, Munro JC, Jones PB *et al.* Schizophrenia and the myth of intellectual decline. *Am J Psychiat* 1997; **154**(5): 635–639.

99. Pidgeon DA. Tests used in the 1954 and 1957 surveys. In: Douglas JWB, editor. *The Home and the School*. London: MacGibbon & Kee, 1964; pp. 129–132.

100. Pidgeon DA. Appendix: details of the fifteen year tests. In: Douglas JWB, Ross JM, Simpson HR, editors. *All Our Futures*. London: Peter Davies, 1968; pp. 194–197.

101. Jones PB. Childhood motor milestones and IQ prior to adult schizophrenia: results from a 43 year old British cohort. *Psychiatria Fennica* 1995; **26**: 63–80.

102. David AS, Malmberg A, Brandt L, Allebeck P, Lewis G. IQ and risk for schizophrenia: a population-based cohort study. *Psychol Med* 1997; **27**(6): 1311–1323.

103. Cannon M, Jones P, Gilvarry K *et al.* Premorbid social functioning in schizophrenia and bipolar disorder: similarities and differences. *Am J Psychiat* 1997; **154**(11): 1544–1550.

104. van Os J, Jones PB, Lewis GH *et al.* Developmental precursors of affective illness in a general population birth cohort. *Arch Gen Psychiat* 1997; **54**: 625–631.

105. Kessler RC, McGonagle KA, Zhao S *et al.* Lifetime and 12-month prevalence of DSM-III-R psychiatric disorders in the United States: results from

the National Comorbidity Survey. *Arch Gen Psychiat* 1994; **52**: 8–19.

106. Mason P, Wilkinson G. The prevalence of psychiatric morbidity. OPCS survey of psychiatric morbidity in Great Britain. *Br J Psychiat* 1996; **168**: 1–3.

107. Office of Population Censuses and Surveys. *OPCS Surveys of Psychiatric Morbidity in Great Britain: Bulletin No. 1. The Prevalence of Psychiatric Morbidity Among Adults Aged 16–64 Living in Private Households in Great Britain*. London: OPCS.

108. Jablensky A, McGrath J, Herrman H *et al*. *National Survey of Mental Health and Wellbeing. Report 4. People Living with Psychotic Illness: An Australian Study*. Australia: Commonwealth of Australia, 1999.

109. Torrey EF, Miller J. *The Invisible Plague. The Rise of Mental Illness from 1750 to the Present*. New Brunswick: Rutgers University Press, 2002; p. 416.

110. Der G, Gupta S, Murray RM. Is schizophrenia disappearing? *Lancet* 1990; **335**: 513–516.

111. Eagles JM, Whalley LJ. Decline in the diagnosis of schizophrenia among first admissions to the Scottish mental hospitals from 1969–78. *Br J Psychiat* 1985; **146**: 151–154.

112. Jones PB, Cannon M. Schizophrenia. In: Martyn CJ, Hughes RAC, editors. *The Epidemiology of Neurological Disorders*. London: BMJ Books, 1997..

113. Harrison G, Owens D, Holton A *et al*. A prospective study of severe mental disorder in Afro-Caribbean patients. *Psychol Med* 1988; **18**: 643–657.

114. Jablensky A, Sartorius N, Ernberg G *et al*. Schizophrenia: manifestation, incidence and course in different cultures. A World Health Organisation ten country study. *Psychol Med* 1992; Monograph Suppl 20.

115. Mortensen PB, Penderson CB, Westergaard T *et al*. Effects of family history and place and season of birth on the risk of schizophrenia. *New Engl J Med* 1999; **340**: 603–608.

116. Pedersen CB, Mortensen PB. Family history, place and season of birth as risk factors for schizophrenia in Denmark: a replication and reanalysis. *Br J Psychiat* 2001; **179**: 46–52.

117. Haukka J, Sivasaari J, Varilo T, Lonnqvist J. Regional variation in the incidence of schizophrenia in Finland: a study of birth cohort born from 1950 to 1969. *Psychol Med* 2001; **31**: 1045–1053.

118. Marcelis M, Takei N, van Os J. Urbanisation and risk for schizophrenia: does the effect operate before or around the time of illness onset? *Psychol Med* 1999: **29**(5): 1197–1203

119. Lewis G, David A, Andreasson S, Allebeck P. Schizophrenia and city life. *Lancet* 1992; **340**: 137–140.

120. Torrey EF, Bowler AE, Clark K. Urban birth and residence as risk factors for psychoses: an analysis of 1880 data. *Schizophrenia Res* 1997; **25**(3): 169–176.

121. Croudace TJ, Kayne R, Jones PB, Harrison GL. Non-linear relationship between an index of social deprivation, psychiatric admission prevalence and the

incidence of psychosis. *Psychol Med* 2000; **30**: 177–185.

122. King M, Coker E, Leavey G *et al*. Incidence of psychotic illness in London: a comparison of ethnic groups. *BMJ* 1994; **309**: 1115–1119.

123. Thomas CS, Stone K, Osborn M *et al*. Psychiatric morbidity and compulsory admission among UK-born Europeans, Afro-Caribbeans and Asians in Central Manchester 1993. *Br J Psychiat* 1993; **163**: 91–99.

124. Wessley S, Castle D, Der G *et al*. Schizophrenia and Afro-Caribbeans. A case-control study. *Br J Psychiat* 1991; **159**: 795–801.

125. Selten JP, Sijben N. First admission rate for schizophrenia in immigrants to The Netherlands: the Dutch National Register. *Soc Psychiat Psychiat Epidemiol* 1994; **29**: 71–72.

126. Burke AW. First admission rates and planning in Jamaica. *Soc Psychiat* 1974; **15**: 17–19.

127. Hickling FW. Psychiatric hospital admission rates in Jamaica, 1971 and 1988. *Br J Psychiat* 1991; **159**: 817–821.

128. Hollister M, Laing P, Mednick SA. Rhesus incompatibility as a risk factor for schizophrenia in male adults. *Arch Gen Psychiat* 1996; **53**: 19–24.

129. McGovern D, Cope RV. First psychiatric admission rate of first and second generation Afro-Caribbeans. *Soc Psychiat* 1987; **22**: 139–149.

130. Warner R. Time trends in schizophrenia: changes in obstetric risk factors with industrialization. *Schizophrenia Bull* 1995; **21**: 483–500.

131. Khoury MJ, Beaty TH, Cohen BH. *Fundamentals of Genetic Epidemiology*. New York: OUP, 1993.

132. Khoury MJ, Beaty TH, Newill CA *et al*. Genetic–environment interactions in chronic airways obstruction. *Am J Epidemiol* 1986; **15**: 65–72.

133. Plomin R, DeFries J, McClearn GI *et al*. *Behvioural Genetics*. New York: Freeman, 2001.

134. Gottesman IJ, Shields J. *Schizophrenia. The Epigenetic Puzzle*. Cambridge: Cambridge University Press, 1982; p. 258.

135. Kendler KS, Diehl SR. Schizophrenia: genetics. In: Kaplan HI, Sadock BJ, editors. *Comprehensive Textbook of Psychiatry VI*, Vol 1. Baltimore: Williams & Wilkins, 1995; pp. 942–957.

136. Kendler KS, McGuire M, Gruenberg AM *et al*. The Roscommon family study. I. Methods, diagnosis of probands and risk of schizophrenia in relatives. *Arch Gen Psychiat* 1993; **50**: 527–540.

137. Kendler KS, McGuire M, Gruenberg AM *et al*. The Roscommon family study. II. The risk of nonschizophrenic, nonaffective psychosis in relatives. *Arch Gen Psychiat* 1993; **50**: 645–652.

138. Kety SS, Wendler PH, Jacobson B *et al*. Mental illness in the biological and adoptive relatives of schizophrenic adoptees. Replication of the Copenhagen study in the rest of Denmark. *Arch Gen Psychiat* 1994; **51**: 442–455.

139. Kety SS. Mental illness in the biological and adoptive relatives of schizophrenic adoptees, findings relevant to genetic and environmental factors in etiology. *Am J Psychiat* 1983; **140**: 720–727.

140. Tienari JP, Wynne CL, Laksy K *et al*. Schizophrenics and their adopted-away offspring. The Finnish adoptive family study of schizophrenia. *Schizophrenia Res* 1997; **24**(1,2): 43.

141. Tienari P. Interaction between genetic vulnerability and family environment: the Finnish adoptive study of schizophrenia. *Acta Psychiat Scand* 1991; **84**: 460–465.

142. Gottesman II, Bertelsen A. Confirming unexpressed genotypes for schizophrenia. Risks in the offspring of Fischer's Danish identical and fraternal twins. *Arch Gen Psychiat* 1989; **46**: 867–872.

143. Jones P, Murray R. The genetics of schizophrenia is the genetics of neurodevelopment. *Br J Psychiat* 1991; **158**: 615–623.

144. Sham P. Genetic epidemiology. *Br Med Bull* 1996; **52**: 408–433.

145. Parnas J, Cannon TD, Jacobsen B *et al*. Lifetime DSM-III-R diagnostic outcomes in the offspring of schizophrenic mothers: results from the Copenhagen high-risk study. *Arch Gen Psychiat* 1993; **50**: 707–714.

146. Kendler KS, McGuire M, Gruemberg AM *et al*. The Roscommon family study. III. Schizophrenia-related personality disorders in relatives. *Arch Gen Psychiat* 1993; **50**: 781–788.

147. Chapman JP, Chapman LJ, Kwapil TR. Scales for the assessment of schizotypy. In: Raine A, Lencz T, Mednick SA, editors. *Schizotypal Personality*. New York: Cambridge University Press, 1995; Chap. 5.

148. Kendler KS, McGuire M, Gruenberg AM *et al*. Schizotypal symptoms and signs in the Roscommon family study: their factor structure and familial relationship with psychotic and affective disorder. *Arch Gen Psychiat* 1995; **52**: 396–403.

149. Cannon TD, Zorrilla LE, Shtasel D *et al*. Neuropsychological functioning in siblings discordant for schizophrenia and healthy volunteers. *Arch Gen Psychiat* 1994; **20**: 89–102.

150. Kendler KS, McGuire M, Gruenberg AM *et al*. The Roscommon family study. IV. Affective illness, anxiety disorders and alcoholism in relatives. *Arch Gen Psychiat* 1993; **50**: 952–960.

151. Crow TJ. The continuum of psychosis and its genetic origins. The sixty-fifth Maudsley lecture. *Br J Psychiat* 1990; **156**: 788–797.

152. Maier W, Lichterman D, Minges J *et al*. Continuity and discontinuity of affective disorders and schizophrenia: results of a controlled family study. *Arch Gen Psychiat* 1993; **50**: 871–883.

153. Squires-Wheeler E, Skodol AE, Bassett A *et al*. DSM-III-R schizotypal personality traits in offspring of schizophrenic disorder, affective disorder, and normal control parents. *J Psychiat Res* 1989; **23**: 229–239.

154. Kidd KK. Can we find genes for schizophrenia? *Am J Med Genet (Neuropsychiat Genet)* 1997; **74**: 104–111.

155. Risch NJ. Linkage strategies for genetically-complex traits. I. Multilocus models. *Am J Hum Genet* 1990; **46**: 222–228.

156. Kidd KK. Associations of disease with genetic markers. Deja vu all over again. *Am J Med Genet (Neuropsychiat Genet)* 1993; **48**: 71–73.

157. Plomin R, Owen MJ, McGuffin P. The genetic basis of complex human behaviours. *Science* 1994; **264**: 1733–1739.

158. Claridge G. Schizotypy and schizophrenia. In: Bebbington P, McGuffin P, editors. *Schizophrenia: The Major Issues.* London: Heinemann, 1988; pp. 187–201.

159. Lewontin RC. The analysis of variance and the analysis of causes. *Am J Hum Genet* 1974; **26**: 400–411.

160. Schizophrenia Linkage Collaborative Group for Chromosomes 3, 6 and 8. Additional support for schizophrenia linkage on chromosomes 6 and 8: a multicenter study. *Am J Med Genet (Neuropsychiat Genet)* 1996; **67**: 580–594.

161. Straub RE, MacLean CJ, O'Neill FA *et al.* A potential vulnerability locus for schizophrenia on chromosome 6p24-22: evidence for genetic heterogeneity. *Nat Genet* 1995; **11**: 287–293.

162. Pulver AE, Lasseter VK, Kasch L *et al.* Schizophrenia: a genome scan targets chromosomes 3p and 8p as potential sites of susceptibility genes. *Am J Hum Genet* 1995; **46**: 222–228.

163. Peltonen L. All out for chromosome 6. *Nature* 1995; **378**: 665–666.

164. Arolt V, Lencer R, Nolte A *et al.* Eye tracking dysfunction is a putative phenotype susceptibility marker of schizophrenia and maps to a locus on chromosome 6p in families with multiple occurrence of the disease. *Am J Med Genet (Neuropsychiat Genet)* 1996; **67**: 580–594.

165. Gill M, Vallada H, Collier D *et al.* A combined analysis of D22S278 markers in affected sib-pairs: support for a susceptibility locus for schizophrenia at chromosome 22q12. *Am J Med Genet (Neuropsychiat Genet)* 1996; **67**: 40–45.

166. Faraone S, Tsuang MT. Methods in psychiatric genetics. In: Tsuang MT, Tohen M, Zahner GEP, editors. *Textbook of Psychiatric Epidemiology.* New York: Wiley-Liss, 1995.

167. Owen M, McGuffin P. DNA and classical genetic markers in schizophrenia. *Eur Arch Psychiat Clin Neurosci* 1991; **240**: 197–203.

168. Wright P, Donaldson PT, Underhill JA *et al.* Genetic association of the HLA DRB1 gene locus on chromosome 6p21.3 with schizophrenia. *Am J Psychiat* 1996; **153**: 1530–1533.

169. Morrison PJ. Anticipating more anticipation. *Lancet* 1996; **347**: 1132.

170. Gorwood P, Leboyer M, Falissard B *et al.* Anticipation in schizophrenia: new light on a controversial problem. *Am J Psychiat* 1996; **153**: 1173–1177.

171. Petronis A, Kennedy JL. Unstable genes, unstable mind. *Am J Psychiat* 1995; **152**: 164–172.

172. Kirov G, Murray R. The molecular genetics of schizophrenia: progress so far. *Molec Med Today* 1997; **March**: 124–129.

173. O'Donovan MC, Guy C, Craddock N *et al*. Expanded CAG repeats in schizophrenia and bipolar disorder. *Nature Genet* 1995; **10**: 380–381.

174. Mimmack ML, Ryan M, Baba H *et al*. Gene expression analysis in schizophrenia: reproducible upregulation of several members of the apolipo-protein L family located in a high susceptibility locus for schizophrenia on chromosome 22. *Proc Natl Acad Sci USA* 2002; **99**(7): 4680–4685.

175. Geddes JR, Lawrie SM. Obstetric complications and schizophrenia: a meta-analysis. *Br J Psychiat* 1995; **167**: 786–793.

176. Lewis SW, Owen MJ, Murray RM. Obstetric complications and schizophrenia: methodology and mechanisms. In: Schultz SC, Tamminga CA, editors. *Schizophrenia: A Scientific Focus*. New York: Oxford University Press, 1989; pp. 56–59.

177. Buka S, Tsuang MT, Lipsitt LP. Pregnancy-delivery complications and psychiatric diagnosis: a prospective study. *Arch Gen Psychiat* 1993; **50**: 151–156.

178. Jones P, Rantakallio P, Hartikainen A-L *et al*. Schizophrenia as a long-term outcome of pregnancy, delivery and perinatal complications: a 28-year follow-up of the 1966 North Finland general population birth cohort. *Am J Psychiat* 1998; **155**(3); 355–364.

179. Kendell RE, Juszczak E, Cole SK. Obstetric complications and schizophrenia: a case-control study based on standardised obstetric records. *Br J Psychiat* 1996; **168**: 556–561.

180. Mednick SA, Machon RA, Huttunen MO *et al*. Adult schizophrenia following prenatal exposure to an influenza epidemic. *Arch Gen Psychiat* 1988; **45**: 171–176.

181. O'Callaghan E, Sham P, Takei N *et al*. Schizophrenia after prenatal exposure to the 1957 A_2 influenza epidemic. *Lancet* 1991; **337**: 1248–1250.

182. Sham PC, O'Callaghan E, Takei N *et al*. Increased risk of schizophrenia following prenatal exposure to influenza. *Br J Psychiat* 1992; **160**: 461–466.

183. Susser E, Lin P. Schizophrenia after prenatal exposure to the Dutch hunger winter of 1944–1945. *Arch Gen Psychiat* 1992; **49**: 983–988.

184. Susser E, Neugebauer R, Hoek HW *et al*. Schizophrenia after prenatal famine: further evidence. *Arch Gen Psychiat* 1996; **53**: 25–31.

185. Huttunen MO, Niskanen P. Prenatal loss of father and psychiatric disorders. *Arch Gen Psychiat* 1978; **35**: 429–431.

186. Myhrman A, Rantakallio P, Isohanni M *et al*. Does unwantedness of a pregnancy predict schizophrenia? *Br J Psychiat* 1996; **169**: 637–640.

187. Rantakallio P, Jones P, Moring J *et al*. Association between central nervous system infections during childhood and adult onset schizophrenia and other psychoses: a 28-year follow-up. *Int J Epidemiol* 1997; **26**(4): 837–843.

188. McGrath JJ, Murray RM. Risk factors for schizophrenia – from conception to birth. In: Hirsch S, Weinberger D, editors. *Schizophrenia*. Oxford: Blackwell, 1995; pp. 187–205.

189. Bracha HS, Torrey EF, Gottesman II *et al*. Second-trimester markers of fetal size in schizophrenia: a study of monozygotic twins. *Am J Psychiat* 1992; **149**: 1355–1361.

190. Davis JO, Bracha HS. Prenatal growth markers in schizophrenia: a monozygotic co-twin control study. *Am J Psychiat* 1996; **153**: 1166–1172.

191. Bradbury TN, Miller GA. Season of birth in schizophrenia: a review of the evidence, methodology and etiology. *Psychol Bull* 1985; **98**: 569–594.

192. Cotter D, Larkin C, Waddington JL *et al*. Season of birth in schizophrenia: clue or cul-de-sac? In: Waddington JL, Buckley PB, editors. *The Neurodevelopmental Basis of Schizophrenia*. RG Landes, 1995.

193. Andreasson S, Allebeck P, Engström A *et al*. Cannabis and schizophrenia. *Lancet* 1987; **2**: 1483–1486.

194. Johnstone EC, Crow TJ, Frith CD, Husband J, Kreel L. Cerebral ventricular size and cognitive impairment in chronic schizophrenia. *Lancet* 1976; **2**: 924–926.

195. Chua SE, McKenna PJ. Schizophrenia – a brain disease?: a critical review of structural and functional cerebral abnormality in the disorder. *Br J Psychiat* 1995; **166**: 563–582.

196. Suddath RL, Christison GW, Torrey EF, Casanova MF, Weinberger DR. Anatomical abnormalities in the brains of monozygotic twins discordant for schizophrenia. *New Engl J Med* 1990; **322**: 789–794.

197. Wright IC, Rabe-Hesketh S, Woodruff PW, David AS, Murray RM, Bullmore ET. Meta-analysis of regional brain volumes in schizophrenia. *Am J Psychiat* 2000; **157**(1): 16–25.

198. McGorry P. Preventative strategies in early psychosis: verging on reality. *Br J Psychiat* 1998; **172**(33): 1–2.

199. Jones P. The new epidemiology of schizophrenia. In: Buckley PF, editor. *Schizophrenia, Psychiatry Clinics of North America*. Philadelphia: WB Saunders, 1998.

200. Warner R. The prevention of schizophrenia: what interventions are safe and effective? *Schizophrenia Bull* 2001; **27**: 551–562.

201. McGlashan TH, Miller TJ, Woods SW. Pre-onset detection and intervention research in schizophrenia psychoses: current estimates of benefit and risks. *Schizophrenia Bull* 2001; **27**: 563–570.

202. Tsuang NT, Storm WS, Sieddman LJ *et al*. Treatment of nonpsychotic relatives of patients with schizophrenia: 4 case studies. *Biol Psychiat* 1999; **45**: 1412–1418.

203. McGorry PD, Yung AR, Philips LJ *et al*. Randomized, controlled trial of interventions designed to reduce the risk of progression to first episode psychosis

in a clinical sample with subthreshold symptoms. *Arch Gen Psychiat* 2002; **59**: 921–928.

204. Lehman AF. Developing an outcomes-oriented approach for the treatment of schizophrenia. *J Clin Psychiat* 1999; **60**: 30–35.

205. Kane JM. Pharmacologic treatment of schizophrenia. *Biol Psychiat* 1999; **46**: 1396–1408.

206. Sartorius N, Fleischhacker WW, Gjerris A *et al*. The usefulness and uses of second generation antipsychotic medications. *Curr Opin Psychiat* 2002; Suppl.

207. Waddington JL, O'Callaghan E. What makes an antipsychotic 'atypical'? Conserving the definition. *CNS Drugs* 1997; **7**: 341–346.

208. Glazer WM. Extrapyramidal side effects, tardive dyskinesia, and the concept of schizophrenia. *J Clin Psychiat* 2000; **61**: 16–21.

209. Ellenbroek BA. Treatment of schizophrenia. A preclinical and clinical evaluation of neuroleptic drugs. *Pharmacol Ther* 1993; **57**: 1–78.

210. Creese I, Burt DR, Snyder S. Dopamine receptor binding predicts clinical and pharmacological properties of antischizophrenic drugs. *Science* 1976; **192**: 481–483.

211. Kapur S, Remmington G. Dopamine D2 receptors and their role in atypical antipsychotic action: still necessary and maybe even sufficient. *Biol Psychiat* 2001; **50**: 873–883.

212. Kapur S, Zipursky R, Remmington G *et al*. Relationship between dopamine D2 occupancy, clinical response, and side effects: a double blind PET study of first episode schizophrenia. *Am J Psychiat* 2000; **157**: 514–520.

213. Kapur S, Zipursky R, Remmington G *et al*. Clinical and therapeutic implications of 5HT2 and D2 receptor occupancy of clozapine, risperidone, and olanzapine in schizophrenia. *Am J Psychiat* 1999; **156**: 286–293.

214. Kapur S, Zipursky R, Remmington G *et al*. PET evidence that loxapine is an equipotent blocker of 5HT2 and receptors: implications for the treatment of schizophrenia. *Am J Psychiat* 1997; **154**: 1525–1529.

215. Xiberas X, Martinot JL, Mallet L, Artiges E *et al*. Extrastriatal and striatal D2 dopamine receptor with haloperidol or new antipsychotic drugs in patients with schizophrenia. *Br J Psychiat* 2001; **179**: 503–508.

216. Allen MH. Managing the agitated psychotic patient: a reappraisal of the evidence. *J Clin Psychiat* 2000; **61**: 11–20.

217. Gilbert G *et al*. Withdrawal of antipsychotic medications. *Arch Gen Psychiat* 2000; **57**.

218. Adams CE, Fenton M, David AS. Systematic meta-review of depot antipsychotic drugs for people with schizophrenia. *Br J Psychiat* 2001; **179**: 290–299.

219. Conley RR, Kelly DL. Management of treatment resistance in schizophrenia. *Biol Psychiat* 2001; **50**: 898–911.

220. Keefe RSE, Silva SG, Perkins DO, Lieberman JA. The effects of atypical antipsychotic drugs on neurocognitive impairment in schizophrenia: a review and meta-analysis. *Schizophrenia Bull* 1999; **25**(2): 201–222.

221. Harvey PD, Keefe RSE. Studies of cognitive change in patients with schizophrenia following treatment with atypical antipsychotics. *Am J Psychiat* 2001; **158**: 176–184.

222. Cunningham-Owens DG. *A Guide to the Extrapyramidal Side Effects of Antipsychotic Drugs*. Cambridge: Cambridge University Press, 1999.

223. Kane JM. Tardive dyskinesia: epidemiological and clinical presentation. In: Bloom FE, Kupfer DJ, editors. *Psychophamracology, A Fourth Generation of Progress*. New York: Raven Press, 1995; pp. 1485–1495.

224. Glazer WM. Expected incidence of tardive dyskinesia associated with typical antipsychotics. *J Clin Psychiat* 2000; **61**: 15–20.

225. Jeste DV. Tardive dyskinesia in older patients. *J Clin Psychiat* 2000; **61**: 27–32.

226. Buckley PF, Adianjee, Sajatovic M. Neuroleptic malignant syndrome. In: Bashir Y *et al*., editors. *Textbook of Neuromuscular Disorders*. Philadelphia: Butterworth-Heinemann, 2001.

227. Arana GW. An overview of side effects caused by typical antipsychotics. *J Clin Psychiat* 2000; **61**: 5–11.

228. Procyshyn R, Thompson D, Tse G. Pharmacoeconomics of clozapine, risperidone, and olanzapine: a review of the literature. *CNS Drugs* 2000; **13**: 47–76.

229. Frangou S, Lewis M. Atypical antipsychotics in ordinary clinical practice: a pharmacoepidemiologic survey in a south London service. *Eur Psychiat* 2000; **15**: 200–226.

230. Geddes J, Freemantle N, Harrison P *et al*. Atypical antipsychotics in the treatment of schizophrenia: systematic overview and regression analysis. *BMJ* 2000; **321**: 1371–1376.

231. Davis JM. Meta-analysis of atypical antipsychotics. Presentation at the Winter Workshop on Schizophrenia Research, Davos, February 2002.

232. Prior C, Clements J, Rowett M *et al*. Atypical antipsychotics in the treatment of schizophrenia [Letter]. *BMJ* 2001; **322**; 324.

233. Glazer WM, Kane JM. Depot neuroleptics therapy: an underutilized treatment option. *J Clin Psychiat* 1992; **53**: 426–430.

234. Richelson E, Souder T. Binding of antipsychotic drugs to human brain receptors – focus on new generation compounds. *Life Sci* 2000; **68**: 29–39.

235. Kane J, Honigfeld G, Singer J *et al*. The Clozapine Collaborative Group. Clozapine for the treatment-resistant schizophrenic: a double-blind comparison with chlorpromazine. *Arch Gen Psychiat* 1988; **45**: 789–796.

236. Rosenheck R, Cramer J, Xu W *et al*. Department of Veterans Affairs Cooperative Study Group of Clozapine in Refractory Schizophrenia. A

comparison of clozapine and haloperidol in hospitalized patients with refractory schizophrenia. *New Engl J Med* 1997; **337**: 809–815.

237. Wallbeck K, Cheine M, Essali A, Adam C. Evidence for clozapine's effectiveness in schizophrenia: a systematic review and metanalysis of randomized trials. *Am J Psychiat* 1999; **156**: 990–999.

238. Chakos M, Lieberman J, Hoffman E. Effectiveness of second-generation antipsychotics in patients with treatment-resistant schizophrenia: a review and meta-analysis of randomized trials. *Am J Psychiat* 2001; **158**: 518–526.

239. Casey DE. Effects of clozapine therapy in schizophrenic individuals at risk for tardive dyskinesia. *J Clin Psychiat* 1998; **59**(3, Suppl): 31–37.

240. Rosenheck R, Dunn L, Peszke M *et al*. Department of Veterans Affairs Cooperative Study Group on Clozapine in Refractory Schizophrenia. Impact of clozapine on negative symptoms and on the deficit syndrome in refractory schizophrenia. *Am J Psychiat* 1999; **156**: 88–93.

241. Walker AM, Lanza L, Arelliano F *et al*. Mortality in current and former users of clozapine. *Epidemiology* 1997; **6**: 671–677.

242. Glazer WM, Dickson RA. Clozapine reduces violence and persistent aggression in schizophrenia. *J Clin Psychiat* 1998; **59**: 8–14.

243. Buckley PF. Substance abuse and schizophrenia: a review. *J Clin Psychiat* 1998, **59**: 26–30.

244. Keefe R, Silva S, Perkins D *et al*. The effects of atypical antipsychotic drugs on neurocognitive impairment in schizophrenia: a review and meta-analysis. *Schizophrenia Bull* 1999; **25**: 201–222.

245. Conley RR. Optimizing treatment with clozapine. *J Clin Psychiat* 1998; **59**(3, Suppl): 44–49.

246. Honigfeld G, Arellano F, Sethi J *et al*. Reducing clozapine-related morbidity and mortality: five years of experience with the Clozaril National Registry. *J Clin Psychiat* 1998; **59**(3, Suppl): 3–7.

247. Kilian J, Kerr K, Lawrence C *et al*. Myocarditis and cardiomyopathy associated with clozapine. *Lancet* 1999; **354**: 1841–1845.

248. Coodin S, Ballegeer T. Clozapine therapy and pulmonary embolism. *Can J Psychiat* 2000; **45**: 395.

249. Allison DB, Mentore JL, Moonseong H *et al*. Antipsychotic-induced weight gain: a comprehensive research synthesis. *Am J Psychiat* 1999; **156**: 1686–1696.

250. Henderson DC, Cagliero E, Gray C *et al*. Clozapine, diabetes mellitus, and weight gain, and lipid abnormalities: a five year naturalistic study. *Am J Psychiat* 2000; **157**: 975–981.

251. Haupt DW, Newcomer JW. Hyperglycemia and antipsychotic medications. *J Clin Psychiat* 2001; **62**: 15–26.

252. Marder SR, Fleishacker WF. Risperidone and olanzapine: experience in clinical practice. In: Buckley PF, Waddington JL, editors. *Schizophrenia and*

Mood Disorders: The New Drug Therapies in Clinical Practice. Bristol: Butterworth-Heinemann, 2000.

253. Keck PE, Wilson DR, Strakowski SM *et al*. Clinical predictors of acute risperidone response in schizophrenia, schizoaffective disorder and psychotic mood disorders. *J Clin Psychiat* 1995; **56**: 466–470.

254. Bouchard R, Merette C, Pourcher E *et al*. Longitudinal comparative study of risperidone and conventional neuroleptics for treating patients with schizophrenia. *J Clin Psychopharmacol* 2000; **20**: 295–304.

255. Green MF, Marshall BD, Wirshing W *et al*. Does risperidone improve verbal working memory in treatment-resistant schizophrenia? *Am J Psychiat* 1997; **154**: 799–804.

256. Chengappa KNR, Sheth S, Brar JS *et al*. A clinical audit of the first 142 patients who received risperidone at a state psychiatric hospital. *J Clin Psychiat* 1999; **60**: 373–378.

257. Currier GW, Simpson GM. Risperidone liquid concentration and oral lorazepam versus intramuscular haloperidol and intramuscular lorazepam for treatment of psychotic agitation. *J Clin Psych* 2001; **62**: 153–157.

258. Emsley RA. Risperidone in the treatment of first-episode psychotic patients: a double-blind multicenter study. *Schizophrenia Bull* 1999; **25**: 721–729.

259. Csernansky JG, Mahmoud R, Brenner R *et al*. The Risperidone User 79 Study Group. A comparison of risperidone and haloperidol for the prevention of relapse in patients with schizophrenia. *New Engl J Med* 2002; **346**: 16–22.

260. Kane JM. Risperidone (Consta) for the treatment of schizophrenia. Presentation at the Winter Workshop on Schizophrenia Research, Davos, February 2002.

261. Bronson B, Lindenmeyer JP. Adverse effects of high-dose olanzapine in treatment-refractory schizophrenia. *J Clin Psychopharmacol* 2000; **20**: 382–384.

262. Tollefson GD, Beasley CM, Tran PV *et al*. Olanzapine versus haloperidol in the treatment of schizophrenia and schizoaffective and schizophreniform disorders: results of an international collaborative trial. *Am J Psychiat* 1997; **154**: 457–465.

263. Tollefson GD, Sanger TM. Negative symptoms: a path analytic approach to a double-blind, placebo- and haloperidol-controlled clinical trial with olanzapine. *Am J Psychiat* 1997; **154**: 466–474.

264. Tollefson GD, Sanger TM, Lu Y *et al*. Depressive signs and symptoms in schizophrenia: a prospective blinded trial of olanzapine and haloperidol. *Arch Gen Psychiat* 1998; **55**: 250–258.

265. Purdon S, Jones B, Stip E. Neuropsychological change in early phase schizophrenia during 12 months of treatment with olanzapine, risperidone, or haloperidol. *Arch Gen Psychiat* 2000; **57**: 249–258.

266. Wright P, Birkett M, David SR *et al*. A double blind placebo controlled comparison of intramuscular olanzapine and intramuscular haloperidol in the treatment of acute agitation in schizophrenia. *Am J Psychiat* 2001; **158**: 1149–1151.

267. Conley RR, Kelly DL, Gale EA. Olanzapine response in treatment refractory patients with a history of substance abuse. *Schizophrenia Res* 1998; **33**: 95–101.

268. Sanger TM, Lieberman JA, Tohen M *et al*. Olanzapine versus haloperidol treatment in first-episode psychosis. *Am J Psychiat* 1999; **156**: 79–87.

269. Tran PV, Dellva MA, Tollefson G *et al*. Oral olanzapine vs oral haloperidol in the maintenance treatment of schizophrenia and related psychoses. *Br J Psychiat* 1998; **172**: 499–505.

270. Lindenmayer JP. Treatment refractory schizophrenia. *Psychiat Quart* 2000; **71**: 373–384.

271. Conley RR, Tamminga CA, Bartko JJ *et al*. Olanzapine compared with chlorpromazine in treatment-resistant schizophrenia. *Am J Psychiat* 1998; **155**: 914–920.

272. Tollefson G, Birkett M, Kiesler G *et al*. Double blind comparison of olanzapine versus clozapine in schizophrenic patients clinically eligible for treatment with clozapine. *Biol Psychiat* 2001; **49**: 52–63.

273. Tollefson GD, Beasley CM, Tamura RN *et al*. Blind, controlled, long-term study of the comparative incidence of treatment-emergent tardive dyskinesia with olanzapine or haloperidol. *Am J Psychiat* 1997; **154**: 1248–1254.

274. Littrell KH, Johnson CG, Littrell S *et al*. Marked reduction of tardive dyskinesia with olanzapine. *Arch Gen Psychiat* 1998; **55**: 279–280.

275. Melkersson K, Hutling A, Brismar K. Elevated levels of insulin, leptin, and blood lipids in olanzapine-treated patients with schizophrenia or related psychoses. *J Clin Psychiat* 2000; **61**: 742–749.

276. Sacchetti E, Guarneri L, Bravi D. H antagonist nizatidine may control olanzapine-associated weight gain in schizophrenic patients. *Biol Psychiat* 2000; **48**: 167–168.

277. Goldstein JM. Quetiapine fumarate (seroquel): a new atypical antipsychotic. *Drugs Today* 1999; **35**(3): 193–210.

278. Kapur S, Zipursky RB, Jones C *et al*. A positron emission tomography study of quetiapine in schizophrenia: a preliminary finding of an antipsychotic effect with only transiently high dopamine D2 receptor occupancy. *Arch Gen Psychiat* 2000; **57**: 553–559.

279. Arvantis LA, Miller BG. Seroquel Trial 12 Study Group. Multiple fixed doses of "Seroquel" (quetiapine) in patients with acute exacerbation of schizophrenia: a comparison with haloperidol and placebo. *Biol Psychiat* 1997; **42**: 233–246.

280. Emsley RA, Raniwalla J, Bailey PJ. On behalf of the PRIZE Study Group. A comparison of the effects of quetiapine (Seroquel) and haloperidol in schizophrenic patients with a history of and a demonstrated partial response to conventional antipsychotic treatment. *Int Clin Psychopharmacol* 2000; **15**: 121–131.

281. Mullen J, Jibson MD, Sweitzer D. A comparison of the relative safety, efficacy and tolerability of quetiapine and risperidone in outpatients with

schizophrenia and other psychotic disorders: the QUEST study. *Clin Ther* 2001; **23**: 1839–1854.

282. Velligan DI, Newcomer J, Peltz J *et al*. Does cognitive function improve quetiapine in comparison with haloperidol. *Schizophrenia Res* 2002; **53**: 239–248.

283. Hellewell JSE, Centillon M, Amermeron Hands D. Seroquel: evidence for efficacy in the treatment of hostility and aggression. *Schizophrenia Res* 1998; **29**: 154–155.

284. Buckley PF, Goldstein J, Emsley RA. Efficacy of quetiapine in patients with poorly responsive schizophrenia. *Schizophrenia Res* 2001; **49**: 221.

285. Glazer WM, Morgenstein H, Pultz J, Yeung PP, Rak IW. Incidence of persistent tardive dyskinesia may be lower with quetiapine treatment than previously reported with typical antipsychotics in patients with psychoses. Presented at American College of Neuropsychopharmacology, Acapulco, Mexico, December 1999.

286. Brecher M, Rak IM, Melvin K, Jones AM. The long-term effects on quetiapine (seroquel) monotherapy on weight in patients with schizophrenia. *Int J Psych Clin Practice* 2001; **4**: 287–291.

287. Potkin SG, Cooper SJ. Ziprasidone and zotepine: clinical experience and use in schizophrenia and mood disorders. In: Buckley PF, Waddington JL, editors. *The New Drug Therapies in Clinical Practice*. Oxford: Arnold, 2000.

288. Keck P, Buffenstein A, Ferguson J *et al*. Ziprasidone Study Group. Ziprasidone 40 mg and 20 mg/day in the acute exacerbation of schizophrenia, and schizoaffecticve disorder: a 4 week placebo controlled trial. *Psychopharmacology* 1998; **140**: 173–184.

289. Brook Slacy JW, Gunn KP for the Ziprasidone IM Study Group. Intramuscular ziprasidone compared with intramuscular haloperidol in the treatment of acute psychosis. *J Clin Psych* 2000; **61**: 933–941.

290. Danials D *et al*. Ziprasidone Switch Study. Presentation at the Annual Meeting of the American Psychiatric Association, New Orleans, 2001.

291. Glassman AH, Bigger JT. Antipsychotic drugs: prolonged qtc interval, torsades de pointes, and sudden death. *Am J Psychiat* 2001; **158**: 1774–1782.

292. Stahl SM. Dopamine system stabilizers, aripiprazole, and the next generation of antipsychotics: "goldilocks" actions at dopamine receptors. *J Clin Psychiat* 2001; **62**: 841–842.

293. Stahl SM. Dopamine system stabilizers, aripiprazole, and the next generation of antipsychotics: illustrating their mechanism of action. *J Clin Psychiat* 2001; **62**: 923–924.

294. Jordan S, Koprivica V, Chen R, Tottori K, Kikuchi T, Altar CA. The antipsychotic aripiprazole is a potent, partial agonist at the human 5HT (1A) receptor. *Eur J Pharmacol* 2002; **441**: 137–140.

295. McQuade R, Burris K, Jordan S, Tottori K, Kurahashi N, Kikuchi T. Aripiprazole: A dopamine-serotonin stabilizer. *Int J Neuropsychopharm* 2002; **5**: S176.

296. Kane JM, Carson WH, Saha AR, McQuade RD, Ingenito G, Zimbroff DL, Aliu M. Efficacy and safety of aripiprazole and haloperidol versus placebo in patients with schizophrenia and schizoaffective disorder. *J Clin Psychiat* 2002; **63**: 763–771.

297. Carson WH, Stock E, Saha AR, Ali M, McQuade RD, Kujawa MJ, Ingenito G. Metaanalysis of efficacy of aripiprazle in the treatment of schizophrenia. *Schizophrenia Res* 2002; **53**: 186.

298. Carson WH, Stock E, Saha AR, Ali M, McQuade RD, Kujawa MJ, Ingenito G. Metaanalysis of safety and tolerability of aripiprazole. *Schizophrenia Res* 2002; **53**: 186–187

299. Buckley PF, Naber D. Quetiapine and sertindole: clinical use and experience. In: Buckley PF, Waddington JL, editors *Schizophrenia and Mood Disorders; the New Drug Therapies in Clinical Practice*. London: Arnold Publications, 2000.

300. Kane JM, Tamminga C. Sertindole (serdolect): preclinical and clinical findings of a new atypical antipsychotic. *Expert Opin Invest Drugs* 1997; **6**: 1729–1741.

301. Zimbroff DL, Kane JM, Tamminga C *et al*. Controlled dose-response study of sertindole and haloperidol in the treatment of schizophrenia. *Am J Psychiat* 1997; **154**: 782–791.

302. Kasper S, Qunier S, Pezawas L. A review of the risk-benefit profile of sertindole. *Int J Psychiat Clin Pract* 1998; **2**: S59–S64.

303. Wilton L, Heeley EL, Pickering RM, Sharkir A. Comparative study of mortality rates and cardiac dysrythmia in post marketing surveillance studies of sertindole and two other atypical antipsychotic drugs, risperidone and olanzapine. *J Psychopharmacol* 2001; **15**: 102–126.

304. Colonna L, Saleem P, Dondey-Nouvel P *et al*. and the Amisulpiride Study Group. Long term safety and efficacy of amisulpiride in subchronic or chronic schizophrenia. *Int Clin Psychopharmacol* 2000; **15**: 13–22.

305. Leucth S, Pitschel-Walz G, Engel RR, Kissling W. Amisulpiride, an unusual 'atypical' antipsychotic: a meta-analysis on randomised controlled trials. *Am J Psychiat* 2002; **159**: 180–190.

306. Cooper SJ, Tweed J, Raniwalla J *et al*. A placebo controlled comparison of zotepine versus chlorpromazine in patients with acute exacerbation of schizophrenia. *Acta Psychiat Scand* 2000; **101**: 218–225.

307. Shiloh R, Zemishlany Z, Aizenberg D *et al*. Sulpiride augmentation in people with schizophrenia partially responsive to clozapine: a double-blind, placebo controlled study. *Br J Psychiat* 1997; **171**: 569–573.

308. Buckley PF, Miller A, Olsen J *et al*. When symptoms persist: clozapine augmentation strategies. *Schizophrenia Bull* 2001; **27**: 615–628.

309. Kupchick M, Spivak B, Mester R *et al*. Combined electroconvulsive–clozapine therapy. *Clin Neuropharmacol* 2000; **23**: 14–16.

310. Lauriello J, Bustillo J, Keith SJ. A critical review of research on psychosocial treatment of schizophrenia. *Biol Psychiat* 1999; **46**: 1409–1417.

311. Bustillo J, Lauriello J, Horan W, Keith SJ. The psychosocial treatment of schizophrenia: an update. *Am J Psychiat* 2001; **158**: 163–175.

312. Fenton WS. Evolving perspectives on individual psychotherapy for schizophrenia. *Schizophrenia Bull* 2000; **26**: 47–72.

313. Hogarty G, Kornblith SJ, Greenwald D *et al*. Three year trials of personal therapy among schizophrenic patients living with or independant of family. *Am J Psychiat* 1997; **154**: 1504–1513.

314. Garety P, Fowler D, Kuipers E. Cognitive-behavioral therapy for medication resistant symptoms. *Schizophrenia Bull* 2000; **26**: 73–86.

315. Dickerson F. Cognitive behavioral psychotherapy for schizophrenia: a review of recent empirical studies. *Schizophrenia Res* 2000; **43**: 71–90.

316. Sensky T, Turkington D, Kingdon D *et al*. A randomized controlled trial of cognitive behavioral therapy for persistant symptoms in schizophrenia resistent to medication. *Arch Gen Psychiat* 2000; **57**: 165–172.

317. Haddock G, Morrison AP, Hopkins R, Lewis S, Tarrier N. Individual cognitive behavioural interventions in early psychosis. *Br J Psychiat* 1998; **172**(Suppl 33): 101–106.

318. Kemp RA, Kirov G, Everitt B, David A. Randomised controlled trial of compliance therapy; 18 month follow up. *Br J Psychiat* 1998; **172**: 413–419.

319. Dixon L, Adams C, Lucksted A. Update on the family psychoeducation of schizophrenia. *Schizophrenia Bull* 2000; **26**: 5–20.

320. Heinssen RK, Liberman RP, Kopelowicz A. Psychosocial skills training for schizophrenia: lessons from the laboratory. *Schizophrenia Bull* 2000; **26**: 21–46.

321. Green MF. Neurocognition and functional outcome. *Schizophrenia Bull* 2000; **26**: 119–136.

322. Thornicroft G, Sczumkler G. *A Textbook of Community Psychiatry*. Oxford: Oxford University Press, 2001.

323. Simmonds S, Coid J, Joseph P *et al*. Community mental health team management in severe mental illness: a systematic review. *Br J Psychiat* 2001; **178**: 497–502.

324. Lehman AF, Goldberg R, Dixon LB *et al*. Improving employment outcomes for persons with severe mental illness. *Arch Gen Psychiat* 2002; **59**: 165–172.

325. Bell M, Bryson G, Greig T *et al*. Neurocognitive enhancement therapy with work therapy. *Arch Gen Psychiat* 2001; **58**: 763–768.

326. O'Reilly R. Involuntary committment. *Psychiat Bull* 2001.

327. Lieberman JA, Perkins D, Belger A *et al*. The early stages of schizophrenia: speculations on the pathogensis, pathophysiology, and therapeutic approaches. *Biol Psychiat* 2001; **50**: 884–897.

328. Tran PV, Hamilton SH, Kuntz AJ *et al*. Double-blind comparison of olanzapine vs risperidone in the treatment of schizophrenia and other psychotic disorders. *J Clin Psychopharmacol* 1997; **17**: 407–418.

329. Bon-Choon H, Miller D, Nopoulos P, Andreasen NC. A comparative effectiveness study of risperidone and olanzapine in the treatment of schizophrenia. *J Clin Psychiat* 1999; **60**: 658–663.

330. Conley RB, Mahmoud R. A randomized double blind study of risperidone and olanzapine in the treatment of schizophrenia or schizoaffective disorder. *Am J Psychiat* 2001; **158**: 1759–1763.

331. Voruganti L, Cortese L, Oyewumi L *et al*. Comparative evaluation of conventional and novel antipsychotic drugs with reference to their subjective tolerability, side-effect profile and impact on quality of life. *Schizophrenia Res* 2000; **43**: 135–145.

332. Blackburn G. Weight gain and antipsychotic medications. *J Clin Psychiat* 2000; **61**: 36–42.

333. Welch R, Chue P. Antipsychotic agents and QT changes. *J Psychiat Neurosci* 2000; **25**: 154–160.

334. Reilly M, Ayis S, Ferrier I *et al*. QTc-interval abnormalities and psychotropic drug therapy in psychiatric patients. *Lancet* 2000; **355**: 1048–1052.

335. Masellis M, Basile V, Ozdemir V *et al*. Pharmacogenetics of antipsychotic treatment: lessons learned from clozapine. *Biol Psychiat* 2000; **47**: 252–266.

336. Fichtner CG, Luchins DJ, Malan RD, Hanrahan P. Real-world pharmacotherapy with novel antipsychotics. *J Pract Psychiat Behav Health* 1999; **5**: 37–43.

337. Weiden PJ, Casey DE. "Polypharmacy": combining antipsychotic medications in the treatment of schizophrenia. *J Pract Psychiat Behav Health* 1999; **5**: 229–233.

338. Kinon BJ, Burson BR, Gilmore JA, Malcom S, Stauffer VL. Strategies for switching from conventional antipsychotic drugs or risperidone to olanzapine. *J Clin Psychiat* 2000; **61**: 833–840.

339. Wirshing DA, Marshall BD, Green MF *et al*. Risperidone in treatment-refractory schizophrenia. *Am J Psychiat* 1999; **156**: 1374–1379.

340. Breier A, Hamilton SH. Comparative efficacy of olanzapine and haloperidol for patients with treatment resistant schizophrenia. *Biol Psychiat* 1999; **45**: 403–411.

341. Conley RR, Tamminga CA, Kelly DL *et al*. Treatment-resistant schizophrenic patients respond to clozapine after olanzapine non-response. *Biol Psychiat* 1999; **46**: 73–77.

342. Evins A, Fitzgerald S, Wine L *et al*. Placebo-controlled trial of glycine added to clozapine in schizophrenia. *Am J Psychiat* 2000; **157**: 826–828.

343. Siris SG, Addington D, Azorin JM *et al*. Depression and management in the USA. *Schizophrenia Res* 2001; **47**: 185–197.

344. Roy A, Thompson R, Kennedy S. Depression in chronic schizophrenia. *Br J Psychiat* 1983; **142**: 465–470.

345. Siris SG. Depression in schizophrenia: perspective in the era of atypical antipsychotic agents. *Am J Psychiat* 2000; **157**: 1379–1389.

346. Buckley PF. Suicide and schizophrenia: effect of clozapine and other atypical antipsychotic medications. *J Crit Illness* 2002; in press.

347. Buckley PF, Noffsinger S *et al*. Violence and schizophrenia. *Psychiat Clin North Am* 2003; in press.

348. Swartz MS, Swanson JW, Hiday VA *et al*. Violence and severe mental illness: the effects of substance abuse and nonadherence to treatment to medication. *Am J Psychiat* 1998; **155**: 226–231.

349. Swartz M, Swenson J, Hiday V *et al*. Randomized, controlled trial of outpatient commitment in North Carolina. *Psych Services* 2001; **52**: 325–329.

350. Drake RE, Mueser KT. Psychosocial approaches to dual diagnosis. *Schizophrenia Bull* 2000; **26**: 105–118.

351. Barraclough C, Haddock G, Tarrier N *et al*. Randomized controlled trial of motivational interviewing, cognitive behavioral therapy, and family intervention for patients with comorbid schizophrenia and substance use disorders. *Am J Psychiat* 2001; **158**: 1706–1713.

352. Buckley PF. Treatment of substance abuse in schizophrenia. *J Clin Psychiat* 1998; **59**: 26–30.

353. Berman I. Obsessive compulsive disorder and schizophrenia. *Psychiat Ann*, Special Issue, 2000.

354. Conley RB. New drugs on the horizon. In: Buckley PF, Waddington JL, editors. *Schizophrenia and Mood Disorders: The New Drug Therapies in Clinical Practice*. Oxford: Arnold, 2001.

355. Mahadik S, Evans D, Khan W *et al*. Phospholipids and the treatment of schizophrenia. *Psychiat Clin North Am* 2003; in press.

356. Arranz M, Munro J, Birkett J *et al*. Pharmacogenetic prediction of clozapine response. *Lancet* 2000; **355**: 1615–1616.

357. Druss BG, Rohrbaugh RM, Levinson CM, Rosenheck RA. Integrated medical care for patients with serious psychiatric illness. *Arch Gen Psychiat* 2001; **58**: 861–868.

358. Drake R, Mueser K, Torrey W *et al*. Evidence-based treatment of schizophrenia. *Curr Psychiat Rep* 2000; **2**: 393–397.

359. Carpenter WT. Evidence-based treatment for first-episode schizophrenia? *Am J Psychiat* 2001; **158**: 1771–1773.

Appendix 1 — Drugs used to treat schizophrenia

Appendix 1

Drug	Trade name	Preparation	Starting dose (mg/day)	Usual dose range for maintenance (mg/day)	Maximum dose (mg/day)
Clozapine	Clozaril Ieponex	Tablet	12.5–25	150–600	900
Risperidone	Risperdal	Tablet, liquid	1–2	3–6	16
Olanzapine	Zyprexa	Tablet, dissolvable wafer	5–10	10–20	20
Quetiapine	Seroquel	Tablet	50–100	300–600	800
Ziprasidone	Geodan	Tablet	40–80	40–160	160
Pimozide	Orap	Tablet	2	2–20	20
Haloperidol	Haldol	Tablet, liquid	1–5	5–25	60
Haloperidol decanoate	Haldol-D	Long-acting injection	25–50 (IM)	50–200/2–4 weeks	300/3–4 weeks
Trifluoperazine	Stelazine	Tablet, liquid	2–5	2–20	20
Zuclopenthixol	Clopixol	Tablet	20–30	20–50	150
Zuclopenthixol deconate	Clopixol-D	Long-acting injection	50–100	200–400/2–4 weeks	600 weekly
Chlorpromazine	Largaltil	Tablet, liquid	50–100	300–800	1000
Thiordazine	Melleril	Tablet, liquid	50–100	300–800	800
Thiothixene	Navane	Tablet, liquid	5–10	15–50	50

Appendix 1

Drug	Trade name	Preparation	Starting dose (mg/day)	Usual dose range for maintenance (mg/day)	Maximum dose (mg/day)
Loxapine	Loxitane	Tablet	20	50–100	150
Perphenazine	Trilafon	Tablet, liquid	4–8	16–56	64
Molindone	Moban	Tablet, liquid	20	50–100	150
Fluphenazine	Prolixin	Tablet, liquid	5	5–20	20
Fluphenazine de canoate	Prolixin D	Long-acting injection	12.5–25	12.5–50/2–4 weeks	100/4 weeks
Zotepine	Zoleptil	Tablet	50–75	150–300	300
Sulpiride	Dolmatil	Tablet	400–800	800–1600	2400
Amisulpiride	Solan	Tablet	400–800	400–800	1200
Aripiprazole	Abilitat	Tablet	15	15–30	30
Sertindole	Serdolect	Tablet	4	12–20	24

(only available in Europe on restricted basis only)

Appendix 2 — Useful Websites

Expert consensus guidelines on schizophrenia
(www.psychguides.com)
Harvard Psychopharmacology Algorithm Project
(www.mhc.com/algorithms)
Medscout: Mental Health
(www.medscout.com/mental_health/index.htm)
Mental Health Infosource
(www.mhsource.com)
(www.mentalhelp.net)
Multimedia medical reference library: psychiatry
(www.med-library.com/medlibrary/Medical_
Reference_Library/Psychiatry)
National Alliance for the Mentally Ill (NAMI)
(www.nami.org)
National Institute for Clinical Excellence
(www.nice.org.uk)
National Institute of Mental Health
(www.nimh.nih.gov/publicat/schizmenu.cfm)
Rethink (National Schizophrenia Fellowship of United
Kingdom)
(www.rethink.org)
SANE
(www.sane.org.uk)
Schizophrenia home page
(www.schizophrenia.com)
WPA site on Stigma Campaign Against Schizophrenia
(www.openthedoors.com)

www.mental-health-matters.com
www.mentalhealth.com
www.mentalwellness.com
www.planetpsych.com
www.psyweb.com

Index

Note: *As schizophrenia is the subject of the book, all index entries refer to schizophrenia unless otherwise indicated. Page numbers followed by 'f' indicate figures; page numbers followed by 't' indicate tables. This index is in letter-by-letter order, whereby spaces and hyphens in main entries are excluded by the alphabetization process. Abbreviations are given in the preface (page v)*